OXFORD MEDICAL PUBLICATIONS

Statistical Questions in Evidence-Based Medicine

D1324564

Statistical Questions in Evidence-Based Medicine

Martin Bland

Professor of Medical Statistics,
St George's Hospital Medical School, London

and

Janet Peacock

Senior Lecturer in Medical Statistics,
St George's Hospital Medical School, London

OXFORD
UNIVERSITY PRESS

OXFORD
UNIVERSITY PRESS

Great Clarendon Street, Oxford OX2 6DP

Oxford University Press is a department of the University of Oxford.
It furthers the University's objective of excellence in research, scholarship,
and education by publishing worldwide in

Oxford New York

Auckland Bangkok Buenos Aires Cape Town Chennai
Dar es Salaam Delhi Hong Kong Istanbul Karachi Kolkata
Kuala Lumpur Madrid Melbourne Mexico City Mumbai Nairobi
São Paulo Shanghai Singapore Taipei Tokyo Toronto

Oxford is a registered trade mark of Oxford University Press
in the UK and in certain other countries

Published in the United States
by Oxford University Press, Inc., New York

First published 2000
Reprinted 2001, 2002 (with corrections), 2004, 2005, 2006, 2008

A catalogue record for this book is available from the British Library

Library of Congress Cataloging in Publication Data
Data available

ISBN 978-0-19-262992-0

7 9 10 8

Typeset by Newgen Imaging Systems (P) Ltd., Chennai
Printed in Great Britain
on acid-free paper by
Biddles Ltd, King's Lynn, Norfolk

For Pauline Bland and Eric Peacock

Preface

For evidence-based practice in medicine, nursing, and allied fields, the practicioner must be able to read the research literature critically. The key skill needed to do this is the ability to understand and interpret statistics. This book is intended to help its readers to do this.

The book began as a course in statistics for medical students. We changed from a lecture-based course to one based on seminars, where students had to read material in advance and prepare the answers to a series of questions. This was a great improvement on our earlier course, the pass rate for our end of year exam rising from 75% to 93%. When a new medical curriculum was introduced this became a course in research and critical skills, concentrating on reading the medical literature, and included not only medical students, but students of biomedical sciences, nursing, physiotherapy, and radiography.

The variety of statistical methods seen in the literature continues to increase, as does the range of statistical knowledge demanded of postgraduate students. We have expanded the book to meet the needs of postgraduate students by including material from our postgraduate teaching. We have indicated questions which we would expect only a graduate student to answer.

The material in the book is drawn entirely from the published literature. Mostly, of course, it is from the medical literature, particularly from those excellent journals the *Lancet* and the *British Medical Journal*. In addition, there are questions drawn from fields allied to medicine and some from the popular media which we thought were relevant or just fun. If the *BMJ* appears to feature rather heavily, this should be taken as tribute to its outstandingly excellent website (www.bmj.com), which we searched often to fill the gaps.

This is a companion volume to Martin Bland's *An Introduction to Medical Statistics* but it will work with any good textbook.

We are very grateful for the critical eyes of our colleagues Barbara Butland and Philip Sedgwick, who read an earlier draft, and to Philip Peacock for his great help in assembling the references. We thank our Japanese translators, Mr K. Adachi and his colleagues, for enabling us to correct several errors. Any errors which remain are, of course, our own, especially as we did our own typesetting (using LATEX) and graphics (using Stata). We also have to thank our ever-supportive head of department, Ross Anderson, to whom we both owe a lot. Most of all, we thank our long-suffering spouses, Pauline and Eric, who we often abandoned (temporarily) in favour of the computer.

Contents

1
Introduction

1.1 Evidence-based medicine

In the early days of medicine, decisions about methods of diagnosis and treatment were based on authority. The opinion of the eminent practitioner, based on experience and the earlier authority of others, was the main source of information. As medicine became more scientific, experience became more formalized, in the form of controlled experiments and formal data collection. Now, doctors are encouraged to use scientific data as the source of their decisions about methods of diagnosis and treatment. We are now in the era of evidence-based medicine. This is a shift in the paradigm of medicine, from authority-based to evidence-based practice. The same process is happening in every field of health-care, so that we now have evidence-based nursing, evidence-based physiotherapy, and so on.

The systematic collection and interpretation of evidence is not new, of course. Doctors such as Pierre–Charles–Alexandre Louis and John Snow were collecting clinical and epidemiological data in middle of the 19th century. Florence Nightingale, 'the Passionate Statistician', regarded statistics as the essential practical tool to prove her points about the health of soldiers and maternity care. It is only in recent years, however, that practice based on systematically collected evidence has become accepted as the standard approach in health-care.

This evidence can be approached by the doctor at various levels. The fundamental level is the paper reporting the results of an individual study. This is important for papers closely related to the doctor's own activity. The next level is the review article, which puts together the evidence and opinion on a topic. Next is the meta-analysis, which combines all the available studies of a topic to give a single estimate of a treatment effect, etc. The Cochrane Collaboration is a worldwide, UK initiated project to provide meta-analyses of all known treatments for all known conditions. It is named after a great UK pioneer of evidence-based medicine, Archie Cochrane. Cochrane Collaboration reviews are updated regularly and distributed in electronic form.

1.2 The role of statistics

Inspection of the research reports in medical journals will show that you need two things to understand a paper. One is a knowledge of the topic being investigated, such as the disease which is being treated, the drugs which are being prescribed, the possible approaches to treatment, etc. The other is an understanding of the research methods being used, the difference between a randomized controlled trial and a case–control study, what is a hazard ratio or a confidence interval, etc. The latter, the collection and interpretation of medical data, comes under the heading of medical statistics. Thus an understanding of statistics is essential for the understanding of medical research.

The central role of statistics is well appreciated in medicine. Not only do all medical students receive an introduction to it, but medical journals such as the *Lancet* and *British Medical Journal* often carry statistical articles. These include series of articles revising basic statistical ideas, such as Statistics Notes in the *British Medical Journal,* and special articles on particular statistical issues, usually concerned with the application of statistical methods to particular medical problems.

1.3 Critical reading

Medical papers are written by fallible human beings like ourselves. Before publication, they are read by referees, usually two. These are experts in the field of the research who comment on the suitability of the paper for publication and suggest improvements to the paper. They are also fallible. There may also be a statistical referee, who is an expert in research methods rather than in the research topic, and is yet another fallible human being. Despite the efforts of authors, their colleagues, referees, and editors, most papers have flaws. These may be in the study design, execution, or interpretation. They may be minor and not affect the conclusions at all, or they may lead the authors into serious error. The reader must beware and should not take any paper at face value. Research must be read critically.

There are good reasons for this. Research in medicine and other health-care fields is largely done by practising clinicians, who also have to attend to the needs of their patients. This is not the way research is done in other fields. Most agricultural research is not done by farmers, for example, but by government-funded research centres and by agrochemical companies such as Zeneca and Monsanto. In most fields research is done by professional researchers. In medical research, many researchers spend only a short period of their careers in research, most of their professional lives being spent in posts where patient care is the principal activity. This has advantages. Most people who will apply the results of research have some experience of the research process. They may therefore have more insight into the difficulties of research and better understanding of its limitations than workers in other disciplines. Their research should be well grounded in practice. The idea that it is one of the duties of health-care professionals to add to knowledge in their field is very attractive. There are serious disadvantages, however. There is a continual flow of inexperienced researchers eager to make their mark. They are seldom well trained in scientific thinking and research methods. They learn on the job and, having learnt, they often leave research forever. Medical research involves many different skills and ways of thinking, and it is impossible for most of us to master all of these. It may be very difficult for medical researchers to get sufficient access to expert advice.

As a result, the medical literature is very prone to error and must be read critically. The purpose of critical reading, also called critical appraisal, is to discover whether the methods used can produce useful information and whether the conclusion drawn by the authors follow from the results of the study.

Medical research is a very difficult business. The essence of research is that we are doing something which has not been done before, and so researchers are bound to make mistakes and not do the best study which is possible with hindsight. Also there are often great limitations in terms of resources, such as the number of patients available, which prevent us doing a flawless study. Researchers are often so close to their project and know it so well that they fail to mention things which are so obvious to them that they forget that the reader does not know them. This may include the purpose of the study! Finally, the pressure on journal space means that information may be omitted which authors would have included if they could. As a result the perfect paper is hard to find and most published research has problems. We should not approach appraisal in a hypercritical, nit-picking way, but in an attempt to make a reasonable judgement on the value of the paper as an addition to knowledge and to decide whether this study is relevant to the question in which we ourselves are interested.

There are useful guidelines to critical reading of the literature (e.g. Sackett *et al.* 1991; Fowkes and Fulton 1991). In this book we concentrate only on the statistical aspects of studies: design, presentation of data, analysis, and interpretation. We have tried to give instant, guided experience, so that our readers will be prepared for many of the difficulties which may be encountered in critical reading.

We have brought together a lot of research from the medical and health-care literature. We have thrown in a few examples from other media as well. The questions vary greatly, from understanding of statistical terms to the detection of quite subtle methodological errors. Research, as we remarked above, is a very difficult business. The researcher is trying to do something no-one has ever done before. Inevitably there are mistakes, which the reader must be able to spot. We hope that the authors whose studies we have used will not be offended by this. We have certainly made a few mistakes ourselves. Those included here, of course, are only the ones we have discovered subsequently.

1.4 How to use this book

The questions are printed on the left-hand page and the answers on the right, so that by concealing the answer page and revealing each answer after considering the question the reader can get instant feedback. Questions which cover material which is not usually part of an undergraduate syllabus in the health sciences are marked with a ✚ in the margin. Questions which are really tricky are marked with a warning ❗.

We have done our best to represent fairly and accurately the studies which we discuss, but it is always possible that we have failed. We have referenced all the studies so the readers can judge for themselves. We have also done our best to give clear, correct answers. Just as we can go wrong in our research, we can go wrong in our critiques. If you find either the question a calumny or the answer obscure, please tell us and we will put it right.

This book is a companion to Martin Bland's *An Introduction to Medical Statistics* and is published simultaneously with the third edition (Bland 2000b). We refer to *An Introduction to Medical Statistics* in many of the answers, so that the reader can get fuller information than we can supply here. Thus *Intro* §7.4 refers to Section 7.4 of the textbook. All the sections in the second edition of *An Introduction to Medical Statistics* are in the third with the same numbers. Where we (rarely) refer to a point not covered in the second edition, we give it as *Intro3* §15.8. The chapters in this book have the same structure as *An Introduction to Medical Statistics*, so that the two books can be used together to form a course. We have also used the same system of identifying material not usually covered in undergraduate courses.

Despite all this, you do not need a copy of *An Introduction to Medical Statistics* to use this book. Any good introductory book on medical statistics will do. (We strongly recommend a book written by a statistician, rather than someone moonlighting from another discipline. You would not want a statistician to remove your appendix, would you?) Each chapter of this book begins with a one-page summary of the material covered, which you can use to find the relevant material in any of the good books now available.

2
The design of experiments

This chapter covers the design of experiments, in particular clinical trials on human patients.

In an experiment or trial we carry out a treatment and observe the outcome. We need a control group who receive no treatment or a different treatment, but are otherwise similar to the group receiving the treatment of interest. The groups of patients should be comparable in every respect except treatment. We achieve this by random allocation, where subjects are allocated to treatments without the subject's own characteristics influencing the choice. Each subject has the same chance of receiving each treatment. Methods to do this include tossing a coin and random number tables.

Experimenters' observations may be influenced by knowledge of which treatment a subject has received. If possible, we should conceal treatment from the observer, a procedure called blinding or masking. Subject response also may be influenced by knowing which treatment they have received, so trial subjects, too, should be blinded if possible. 'Double-blind' means that neither the subject nor the experimenter knows the treatment allocation. Where there is no control treatment, we may use a 'placebo', which is an inactive treatment, outwardly as similar as possible to the active treatment.

A cross-over trial is one where each subject receives all treatments, in random order. Each subject acts as their own control. This is good for treatments which control symptoms in chronic disease. We need a smaller sample size than for a two-sample trial, but we cannot look at long-term effects of treatments or at treatments which cure the disease.

Treatment groups are comparable at randomization, but this may change if some patients drop out or switch treatments. To keep the groups comparable, we analyse according to the original intention to treat, including everybody as if they had received the treatment to which they were allocated, whether they actually did or not.

Sometimes trial subjects are allocated into treatments in clusters, e.g. all patients in a general practice. The cluster is the experimental unit. Data must be analysed in experimental units, not as individual subjects.

It is essential that trials on human subjects be carried out ethically, the welfare of the trial subject being the researchers' primary concern. Potential subjects should be informed as fully as possible of what is involved in the trial and their free consent obtained.

QUESTIONS

2.1   Following a heart attack, patients are often prescribed drugs to prevent further attacks. An audit was done to look at the effect of introducing a simple intervention to advise the general physician of the recommended treatment regime (aspirin + another drug). The authors compared patterns of drug prescribing among patients discharged before and after the introduction of the scheme (Smith and Channer 1995).

2.1.1   What comparison is being made in this study?

2.1.2   How might the study design affect the interpretation of results here?

2.1.3   Suggest another study design to look at the effects of this intervention. What would be the problems with this?

2.2   To evaluate a campaign advertising the main symptoms of diabetes, three random samples of the general public were interviewed: the first before the campaign, the second at the end of, and the third 10 weeks after. Their knowledge of the symptoms of diabetes was recorded. No subject was questioned on more than one occasion (Singh *et al.* 1994).

2.2.1   Which groups are being compared in this study?

2.2.2   What are the difficulties in interpreting results from this study?

2.2.3   Are any other approaches feasible?

2.3   Phase 3 of the NHS and Community Care Act, which transferred some responsibility for the care of elderly patients from the National Health Service to local government, was implemented on 1 April 1993. To investigate the effect of this on hospital practice, patients aged 65+ in one hospital between 1 April 1992 and 31 March 1994 were studied. Two groups of randomly selected patients were compared: 100 discharged before 1 April 1993 and 100 discharged after. Most hospital staff were unaware of the monitoring and the decision to discharge was taken by ward staff and not by investigators. Outcomes recorded included the number of days in hospital and whether discharge was within 10 days of becoming medically stable (Ajayi *et al.* 1995).

2.3.1   Why might the investigators think it important that discharge was decided by staff who were unaware of the investigation?

2.3.2   Despite this, what biases might affect the study's findings?

ANSWERS

2.1.1   This study compares prescribing practice before and after guidelines were introduced.

2.1.2   These are historical not concurrent controls. Any change in prescribing could be due to other factors which occurred or changed in that time period. These could include media attention to the subject, patient demand, the introduction of other guidelines, etc. (*Intro* §2.1).

2.1.3   The gold standard for testing an intervention is the randomized controlled trial. In this design the intervention group would be compared with a concurrent control group and the allocation to groups would be done at random. There are some difficulties with such a study such as the reluctance to withhold the intervention, contamination of intervention and control groups—physicians talk to each other (*Intro* §2.2).

2.2.1   Random samples of people at three points in time—before, just after and 10 weeks after an advertising campaign—were compared to see if their knowledge of the symptoms of diabetes had changed. The comparison between the group just after the campaign and the group at 10 weeks looked for evidence that any change observed just after the campaign was sustained.

2.2.2   Other events happening at the same time as the campaign may have affected knowledge, so it is difficult to separate out the effects of the campaign itself (*Intro* §2.1).

2.2.3   A randomized trial at the individual level would be impossible because contact among the subjects might contaminate the non-intervention group. A randomized trial where different areas received publicity or no publicity would be difficult because it would need a large number of areas. Contamination could also be a problem as individuals in areas receiving no publicity might still obtain it by other means (media, friends, etc.). This might reduce the apparent difference between people exposed to and not exposed to the campaign.

2.3.1   It is likely that the investigators will have views on the act and its effects on discharge. If they were deciding on the discharge, they may be influenced in their decision by their desired research outcome. Being aware of this problem might lead them to be biased in the other direction. They therefore monitored discharges decided on by others. If the staff making the discharge decision were aware of the investigation, they might be biased in the same way.

2.3.2   Other secular changes in the 2-year interval apart from the introduction of the act, might lead to a change in hospital practice. Events such as hospital/ward closures, change in case-mix, etc. might explain any changes observed (*Intro* §2.1).

QUESTIONS

2.4   In a study of birth position in labour, 218 women were randomly allocated to squatting using a birth cushion and 209 to conventional management. Fourteen percent of women did not use the position to which they had been allocated. The two groups were compared according to the original intention to treat, irrespective of the posture adopted. The squatting group had fewer forceps deliveries and shorter mean duration of labour (Gardosi *et al.* 1989).

2.4.1   What is meant by 'randomly allocated'? Why was this done?

2.4.2   Why were the groups analysed according to the original intention to treat?

2.4.3   Why is it impossible to have blind assessment in this trial and does this matter?

2.5   Second-line drugs in the treatment of rheumatoid arthritis are prescribed to reduce the risk of flare-up of the disease. Their effectiveness had been established in short-term studies. A study was done to see whether patients who have responded to such drugs benefit from long-term use. In a 52-week double-blind trial, 285 patients who were taking second-line drugs were randomized to continue the therapy or to placebo. At 52 weeks, a flare had occurred in 38% of the placebo group compared with 22% of the continued therapy group (ten Wolde *et al.* 1996).

2.5.1   What is meant by 'placebo' and why was this used here?

2.5.2   What is meant by 'double-blind' and why was this done?

ANSWERS

2.4.1 Randomly allocated means that the choice of management does not depend on any characteristics of the women themselves. Each woman has an equal chance of being allocated to either conventional management or squatting. Random allocation can be done by tossing a coin, by using random number tables, or a similar method. Because the allocation is at random, the two groups will be comparable apart from the treatment and so any differences in outcome between the groups could be attributed to the differences in management (*Intro* §2.2).

2.4.2 Randomization produces groups which are comparable apart from the treatment. If the groups are analysed according to the original intention to treat, the comparability of the groups is maintained. This means that even if subjects do not adopt the allocated birth position throughout, they are still analysed as if they did. The alternative would be to either omit non-compliers or to put them into the group according to how they actually delivered. This should not be done as non-compliers are likely to be different to the rest of the sample and so the balance of the groups would be upset and bias introduced (*Intro* §2.5).

2.4.3 The two birth positions are different and women would know which they had been allocated to. Hence they could not be blind. The obstetrician or midwife would be able to see which group the women was allocated to and so could not be blind either. This might affect the management of the labour such as the decision to use forceps (*Intro* §2.8, 2.9).

2.5.1 A placebo is an inert treatment used when there is no alternative treatment for the control group. It is used so that the subjects do not know whether they are receiving the active treatment or the control. It is particularly important when subjective measurements are being made. If the subjects knew which treatment they were receiving, it might affect their reporting of a flare due to psychological effects. The knowledge that a subject has been given a treatment to reduce flare-ups may itself reduce flare-ups, or lead the subjects to think that they experience a reduction. They may also report fewer flare-ups as they know this is what the doctor wants to hear.

2.5.2 If the subjects do not know which treatment they receive, they are said to be blind to the treatment. Knowledge of the patients' treatment may also affect the researcher making the assessment of the patients' condition and so it is desirable that observers do not know the treatment either. In this case assessment is blind. A trial where both subjects and assessors are blind is called a double-blind trial (*Intro* §2.8, 2.9).

QUESTIONS

2.6   In an experiment investigating the effectiveness of topical analgesia prior to venepuncture, 35 volunteer subjects each acted as their own controls. They were given a treatment, active (EMLA) or placebo on one arm. The outcome measure was the time taken for the area of application on the arm to go numb. This was then repeated for placebo or treatment on the other arm. The choice of treatment for each arm and the order of application were both random (Nott *et al.* 1996).

2.6.1   Explain what 'random' means in this context and why it was done.

2.6.2   What are the advantages of this study design and what are the implications for the statistical analysis.

2.7   To study the use of aspirin in the prevention of heart disease and stroke, 5 139 doctors were randomly allocated to either a treatment group who took 500 mg aspirin daily or a control group who were given no treatment. The subjects completed a short health questionnaire every 6 months for 6 years and certificates were obtained for all deaths. Reports of disease from questionnaires were classified by blind assessors (Peto *et al.* 1988).

2.7.1   What is a 'blind assessor'?

2.7.2   Was this trial double-blind?

2.7.3   How would the trial design influence the interpretation of a difference in total mortality?

2.7.4   How would the trial design influence the interpretation of a difference in the number of attacks of migraine reported between the treatment and control groups? (This was a secondary outcome.)

❶ 2.7.5   Do you think that there is anything about this trial which might make a placebo ineffective?

2.8   In a study of two antibiotics to treat chlamydia among pregnant women, erythromycin (500 mg four times daily) was compared to amoxycillin (500 mg three times daily). The drugs were issued in identical capsules in blister packs. For amoxycillin, there were four doses each day, the third one being a placebo. Women were randomly assigned to treatment (Alary *et al.* 1994).

❶   Why was one of the four daily doses a placebo in this trial?

ANSWERS

2.6.1   There are two elements of randomness in this study. First the choice of treatment for each arm was random, i.e. there was an equal chance that an arm was given the treatment or placebo. This means that the characteristics of the subject such as handedness did not affect which treatment was given to each arm. In addition, since each arm was assessed separately the order of assessment was random so that any effect of ordering is removed.

2.6.2   The advantage of this design is that the two treatments are compared within subjects. This removes the effects of differences between subjects and thus is a more powerful design. To take advantage of this design, the analysis will need to be done within subjects too, i.e. the outcome will be the differences within subjects in time to numbness for the two arms.

2.7.1   A blind assessor does not know which treatment each subject is receiving. This is important as the assessment of a treatment may be biased by a desire for success, particularly in the case of a subjective measurement as here. The classification of diseases from written reports clearly requires judgement.

2.7.2   In a double-blind trial neither the subject nor the assessor knows which treatment he is receiving. The subjects knew which group they were in, so the trial is not double-blind (*Intro* §2.9).

2.7.3   The lack of blindness is unlikely to affect total mortality as it is not a subjective outcome. There could be some impact on other behaviour such as risk taking, but it seems unlikely that this would have a major impact. (*Intro* §2.8).

2.7.4   Reporting of migraine is subjective and it may be associated with the treatment in subjects' minds. Hence, this could lead to a reduction of reported attacks in the treated group (*Intro* §2.8).

2.7.5   The subjects were doctors and so would find it very easy to discover whether their tablets actually contained aspirin (*Intro* §2.9).

2.8   One dose was a placebo because the number of active doses was different for the two treatments. Including a dummy dose made the number the same so that the treatment could be concealed (*Intro* §2.8).

QUESTIONS

2.9   Two treatments used to stop breast milk secretion were compared. One
was bromocriptine twice daily for 14 days, the other was a single dose
of cabergoline. Two hundred and seventy-two women were randomized
to two equal sized groups. One group received a placebo after delivery
and two doses of bromocriptine each day for 14 days, the other received
a dose of cabergoline after delivery and a placebo twice daily for 14 days
(Anonymous 1991).

Why was each woman given a placebo treatment?

2.10   Two randomized controlled trials comparing routine ultrasonography
screening during pregnancy with no ultrasound screening were carried
out, to see whether routine ultrasound imaging influenced outcomes of
pregnancy such as birthweight and mode of delivery. To study possible
long-term effects of ultrasonography, at ages 8–9 years, 2 011 singleton
children of women who had taken part in these trials were followed
up and their educational attainment measured. Ultrasonography had
actually been carried out on 92% of the 'screened' group and 5% of the
control group. Analysis was by intention to treat (Salvesen et al. 1992).

What might be the effect on the results of some of the controls receiving
ultrasound examinations and some of the 'screened group' not being
scanned?

2.11   In a trial of the treatment of chronic fatigue syndrome, 60 patients
were allocated randomly to standard medical treatment or standard
medical treatment plus cognitive behaviour therapy. Three patients
randomized to medical care only did in fact receive psychotherapy in
addition, and one patient allocated to cognitive behaviour therapy also
received counselling. An intention to treat analysis showed that 73% of
cognitive therapy patients achieved a satisfactory outcome, compared
to 27% of patients given medical care only (Sharpe et al. 1996).

What effect might the extra psychotherapy have on the results?

ANSWERS

2.9   The treatments were very different in administration, so although each woman received an active treatment she was given a dummy of the other treatment so that she would not know which she had received. This is sometimes known as a double-dummy (*Intro* §2.8).

2.10   Women given ultrasound who were not originally allocated to it may have had a high-risk pregnancy. Women who were not given ultrasound despite being allocated to it may be likely to refuse any medical advice, not just ultrasound, and so may have worse health. Only if we analyse according to intention to treat will we have comparable groups. If we analyse by actual treatment, the ultrasound group may contain subjects who are at high risk for medical reasons and the no ultrasound group subjects at high risk for social reasons. Either of these may lead to differences in attainment, in either direction. On the other hand, if there are no such selection effects, intention to treat analysis may dilute the effect of the ultrasound (*Intro* §2.5).

2.11   The two treatment groups should be comparable at the start, because they are randomized. However, three patients allocated to medical care only also received psychotherapy. If the extra psychotherapy were effective, this might reduce the difference between the groups slightly and so bias the estimated difference downwards towards zero. If the extra counselling for a member of the treatment group were effective, this might increase the difference (*Intro* §2.5).

QUESTIONS

2.12 In an attempt to prevent further cardiac events (heart attack, need for by-pass surgery, sudden death) 468 survivors of heart attacks were allocated randomly to receive daily tablets of magnesium hydroxide or placebo for 1 year. There was a slight excess of adverse events in the treatment group compared with the placebo group but this was not statistically significant. For patients who kept to the treatment, there was a larger and statistically significant excess risk of a cardiac event for the magnesium group compared to the control group (Galloe *et al.* 1993).

 Two analyses were presented, one according to the intention to treat and the other excluding drop-outs. What are the implications of the two analyses and is the approach justified?

2.13 A randomized, double-blind, placebo-controlled cross-over study investigated the effect of alcohol consumption on hormone levels. The intervention was to drink a given measure of alcohol on one day and a placebo drink on the other with the order being randomized. The outcome measure for each woman was the difference in the level of hormones (oestradiol and oestrone) in the blood for the alcohol and placebo days (Ginsburg *et al.* 1996).

2.13.1 What is meant by a 'cross-over' study?

2.13.2 Why was the order of drinks randomized?

2.13.3 What are the advantages of this design compared to randomization to an alcohol group and a placebo group?

2.14 Nine hundred and eighty patients fitted with permanent cardiac pacemakers were included in a study of interference with pace-makers by cellular telephones. Five types of hand-held telephone were tested on each patient in random order. Patients were electrocardiographically monitored while the telephones were being tested to assess any interference with normal cardiac rhythm. Two tests were used per telephone and each patient was allowed a recovery period between tests (Hayes *et al.* 1997).

2.14.1 Why were the five telephones tested on each patient?

2.14.2 Why were patients allowed a recovery period between tests?

ANSWERS

2.12   The first analysis compares the groups as they were originally allocated at random and so any differences could be attributed to the treatment. This analysis suggested a possible harmful effect of magnesium but was consistent with no difference between the treatments. When patients who dropped out were excluded, there was a statistically significant excess risk of a cardiac event in the magnesium group. In this case the secondary analysis excluding drop-outs was done to ensure that a harmful effect of magnesium was not missed and may be justified (*Intro* §2.5).

2.13.1   In a cross-over study each subject acts as their own control and so the effect of alcohol on hormone levels is measured within women. It is possible here because the effect of alcohol on hormone level is of short duration (*Intro* §2.6).

2.13.2   The order of drinks was randomized because the order of consumption might affect the outcome. In addition randomization makes it possible for the women to be blind to which drink they are receiving.

2.13.3   The advantage of this design is that the effects of alcohol are assessed within women rather than between women which would be the case if one group were given alcohol and another were given placebo. The cross-over design thus removes variation between women in the assessment of effects of alcohol and leads to a more precise overall estimate of the effect (*Intro* §2.6).

2.14.1   Cardiac function varies from patient to patient. If the five telephones were given to five different groups of patients, then the precision of differences between the telephones would be reduced by random variation between the patients. By comparing the telephones within patients, a cross-over design, the between patient variability is removed and the effects can be estimated within patients with higher precision.

2.14.2   Patients were allowed a recovery period so that if there was any interference with cardiac rhythm, then the heart would have time to regain its normal rhythm before the next test began (*Intro* §2.6).

QUESTIONS

2.15   During a feverish illness, young children may sometimes have a febrile convulsion, a fit similar to an epileptic fit. Febrile convulsions are very frightening to parents, but they do not mean that the child is epileptic. They sometimes recur. Wallace and Smith (1980) carried out a study to see whether treating children with one of two anti-epileptic drugs, phenobarbitone or valproic acid, would reduce the risk of further convulsions.

The subjects in this trial were 121 children who had had their first convulsions during a feverish illness of 38°C or more, and were consecutive admissions to five paediatric units. Children were thought to be at increased risk of another fit if they were young (under 19 months), had an abnormal neurological state, had a family history of seizures, or the initial convulsion was multiple, prolonged, or on one side of the body only. Parents of these high-risk children were advised alternately to give either phenobarbitone or valproic acid. Low-risk children were prescribed either phenobarbitone, or valproic acid, or no treatment. Allocation was sequential.

2.15.1   Was the original allocation scheme reasonable? Why were children split into high- and low-risk groups?

Things started to go wrong. Many parents could not be persuaded that their child should be given the drugs, even though they were in the high-risk group. The authors decided to reclassify the children into three groups: receiving phenobarbitone (as allocated), receiving valproic acid (as allocated), or receiving no treatment (as allocated or because parents refused). The distinction between high- and low-risk was abandoned. Despite this parental refusal, 117 of the 121 children were followed for at least 2 years, an exceptionally high follow-up.

2.15.2   What method was used to deal with the failure of the subjects to comply? What did this do to the composition of the groups used in the analysis?

Blood levels of the drugs were measured every 6 months. Episodes of feverish illness were recorded from parents' reports as definite illnesses requiring the intervention of a doctor or a temperature of 38°C. All fits were recorded.

2.15.3   What method of ascertainment of feverish illness was used? Could this lead to bias in data collection?

ANSWERS

2.15.1   Children were divided into two groups on the basis of pre-determined risk factors, to give a high- and a low-risk group. The high-risk group were then allocated alternately to phenobarbitone or valproic acid. This means that the first was prescribed phenobarbitone, the second valproic acid, the third phenobarbitone, the fourth valproic acid, and so on. The low-risk group was prescribed sequentially phenobarbitone, valproic acid, and nothing. It would be better to randomize, because then the trial could be blind, but there is no reason to suppose that any bias would occur. We could analyse it simply as two separate trials, one in high-risk and another in low-risk children. The main problem with alternate allocation is that the doctor knows to what treatment the child will be allocated when recruiting it to the trial. The authors do not say why they split the children into high- and low-risk groups, but a possible reason was that they thought it unethical not to offer treatment to the children they thought to be at high risk.

2.15.2   The authors assumed that those who refused the treatment were comparable to those who accepted it, and placed the refusals in the control group. This means that we cannot distinguish between the effects of the treatment and the effects of differences in health behaviour, etc., between the groups. Refusals in trials usually have a worse prognosis than acceptors, and we may have a control group that is likely to have more fits than the treated groups, irrespective of treatment. We must analyse the data by the intention to treat if we are to have comparable groups.

2.15.3   Parents determined the child's temperature to be over 38°C and decided whether the doctor was needed. Whether they are likely to call the doctor for minor symptoms, and whether they are able to measure the child's temperature or are interested in doing so, will depend on their general health behaviour and may be related to whether they accept treatment for their child. Thus there may be more feverish episodes of a less severe nature among the treated children than among the controls.

QUESTIONS

For the analysis, only those 6-month periods of follow-up when the child had a feverish illness were used. These periods were categorized as the child receiving no treatment, optimum doses of phenobarbitone or valproic acid as determined by the blood measurements, or sub-optimal doses of phenobarbitone or valproic acid. The presence or absence of fits in these 6-month periods was noted. This produced the following results:

Febrile convulsions in children studied for 6-month periods

	Fits	No fits	% Periods with fits
Phenobarbitone (optimum)	6	39	13
Phenobarbitone (sub-optimum)	8	50	14
Valproic acid (optimum)	5	34	13
Valproic acid (sub-optimum)	6	29	17
No drug treatment	34	66	34

! 2.15.4   What was the experimental unit? How should this have affected the analysis?

Fits were twice as frequent in the no drug periods as in the drug treatment periods, which were all very similar. The no drug periods versus drug periods comparisons were all statistically significant.

The authors suggested that the reason for the lack of difference between the optimum and sub-optimum drug periods was because parents who complied to some extent with the treatment were better at using other methods of reducing risk during fever. These include cooling the child physically by removing clothing, sponging with warm water, and lowering the room temperature, and by giving paracetomol or aspirin.

! 2.15.5   If the untreated children had more fits, why was this?

2.15.6   How could the design of this study have been improved?

ANSWERS

2.15.4   The child was allocated to treatment so the child is the experimental unit, not the 6-month period. The data should have been presented in terms of percentage of children who had fits, or average number of fits experienced by a child. If there were a difference in the severity of the febrile illnesses (and thus in the risk of a fit) between the groups, this might affect the frequencies in the 'No fits' column and so bias the percentage, because only periods with feverish illness requiring medical intervention were used.

2.15.5   We cannot say why untreated children appear to have had more fits. It could be the treatment; it could be other differences. For example, the parents of the treated children could be better at other health measures such as physical cooling and aspirin.

2.15.6   This would have been much better as a randomized double-blind placebo controlled trial design. The outcome would be whether or not the child had a fit, or the number of fits per year, the unit of analysis being the child. Then the only children in the trial would be those whose parents agreed to the treatment of their children. They should be comparable in their use of other cooling measures. They might subsequently change their minds, and this would be dealt with by analysis by intention to treat.

QUESTIONS

2.16 A study was carried out in Nepal to assess the effects of two vitamin supplementation regimes, continuous, weekly, low dose supplementation of vitamin A or provitamin A (β carotene) on mortality related to pregnancy in women of reproductive age. Sample size calculations suggested that about 7 000 pregnancies would be required in each of the two treatment groups and in a placebo group. A total of 270 electoral wards in 30 sub-districts (nine wards each) covering an area of around 500 km^2 with a total population of around 176 000 participated in the study. At a local crude birth rate of 41 per 1 000 population per year, the authors anticipated that recruiting 21 000 pregnancies would take around 3 years.

All wards were assigned by a random draw of numbered chits, blocked on sub-district, for eligible women to receive one of three apparently identical coded dietary supplements. These were opaque, gelatinous capsules containing peanut oil and preformed vitamin A, β carotene, or no vitamin A or β carotene (placebo). Mortality rates were 704 per 100 000 pregnancies in the placebo group, 426 in the vitamin A group, and 361 in the β carotene group (West *et al.* 1999).

➕ 2.16.1 What type of randomized trial is this?

❗➕ 2.16.2 What effect does this design have on the analysis?

➕ 2.16.3 What is meant by 'blocked on sub-district'? Why was this done?

ANSWERS

2.16.1   This is a cluster-randomized trial, the women in an electoral ward form-
         ing a cluster (*Intro* §2.11).

2.16.2   The effect of the cluster randomization is to make the women in a treat-
         ment group more like one another than they would be if each woman
         was randomized individually. This must be allowed for in the analysis,
         making the confidence intervals wider than they would be if the cluster-
         ing were ignored. The authors of this paper did this (*Intro* §2.11, *Intro3*
         §10.13).

2.16.3   Within each sub-district there are nine wards. The randomization was
         done so that in each sub-district three wards were allocated to each
         treatment. This reduced the possible effects of geographical differences
         between the treatment groups (*Intro* §2.2).

3
Sampling and observational studies

There are many possible designs for observational studies, where no intervention or treatment takes place.

A census is a count of a population, where every member of the population is studied. For many purposes this is impractical so we use a sample. We want the sample to be representative, i.e. to have the same characteristics as the population. To achieve representativeness, we must not allow the subjects' own characteristics to affect whether they are included in the sample. We allow chance to select the sample, giving each subject the same probability of being selected. We can use random number tables to do this. We need a sampling frame, a list of the population, from which to sample. In medical research access to subjects is often difficult and several different, non-random designs are used.

In a cross-sectional study, we take a group of subjects, observe them once, and look at relationships between the variables we observe.

A cohort study follows a group of subjects over time, observing them at least twice. We see whether observations made at the start, often possible risk factors, can predict observations at the end, often the occurrence of disease. The design has the advantages that information on the risk factor is collected 'blind' to the outcome, and risk and relative risk can be calculated directly. Recall bias is avoided. Disadvantages are that it takes a long time, requires a relatively large sample, and is expensive. For rare diseases a very large sample and long follow-up is needed.

In a case–control study, we compare a group of subjects with a disease, the cases, with a group without the disease, the controls. This design is used in clinical research to study the natural history of disease and in epidemiology to study its possible causes. Compared to a cohort study, the design gives a quicker answer with a smaller sample. It can be used with rare diseases without needing a very large sample. The disadvantages are that the control group may not be comparable with the cases, data collection often relies on memory which may be influenced by the disease (recall bias), information may be poor because we rely on memory of past events, cases may have been detected because of medical examinations connected with the risk factor (detection bias), interviewers may be aware of whether the subject is a case and so be biased (assessment bias).

An ecological study is one where variables are collected not on individuals but on populations. We must be very wary of inferring a relationship at the individual level.

QUESTIONS

3.1   In a study of psychological function in dialysis patients, 27 randomly selected patients were matched for age and IQ to healthy volunteer subjects (Altmann *et al.* 1989). Results for accuracy and time taken in a test of visual spatial ability are shown below:

	Accuracy	Time (s)
Patients		
Mean	24.7	13.8
Standard error	1.1	1.3
Controls		
Mean	28.7	13.6
Standard error	0.7	1.2

3.1.1   What is meant by randomly selected and why was this done?

3.1.2   What is meant by matched?

3.1.3   Why do you think this design might have been adopted?

3.2   Questionnaires were sent to a random sample of 200 GPs in East Anglia, asking about their diagnosis and treatment of hypertension. Replies were received from 125. GPs were asked what was the minimum blood pressure they would regard as showing hypertension, and which was the minimum pressure at which they would begin treatment. The study found that the cut-off above which treatment would be given was higher than that used for diagnosis (Dickerson and Brown 1995).

3.2.1   What is meant by a random sample and how might it be chosen?

3.2.2   Why was a random sample used here?

3.2.3   How might the response rate affect the findings?

ANSWERS

3.1.1   Randomly selected means the patients are a random sample of some larger population. The sample is chosen so as to give each member of the population the same probability of being chosen. It is done to obtain a representative sample of the patients so that the results of the study can be generalized to the larger population (*Intro* §3.4).

3.1.2   Matched means that for each patient a healthy volunteer of the same age and IQ, within pre-specified limits, was chosen. This means that differences in age and IQ will not produce difference in test score between the groups (*Intro* §3.8).

3.1.3   IQ is an important factor influencing performance on psychological test. However, it is time consuming to measure and the researchers are unlikely to have tested a large number of normal subjects to find matches. If the researchers had available a database of test results on normal subjects, however, this design is efficient, because they could choose their matched controls from this database.

3.2.1   A random sample is a group of subjects taken from a larger population so that each member of the population has an equal chance of being selected. The characteristics of the subject do not influence the chance of being chosen. This can be done using random number tables, computer generated random numbers, etc. (*Intro* §3.4).

3.2.2   It is done so that the sample will be representative of the population and we can use the sample to tell us about the population. Here, the replies of the sample will provide information about the views of all GPs in East Anglia, without the expense of asking them (*Intro* §3.4).

3.2.3   The response rate was 63% which is quite low, although not unusual in general practice research. It is possible that GPs who replied to the survey were different from those who did not in ways which were related to the treatment of high blood pressure. Hence, the sample may not be representative of all GPs.

QUESTIONS

3.3   It has been suggested that reducing serum cholesterol may increase the
risk of death from accident, poisoning or violence. This was investigated
using a random sample of people born between 1913 and 1947 and living in North Karalla, Finland. During the 1970s, serum cholesterol was
measured for each subject. All deaths from accident, poisoning or violence from this time to 1987 were obtained from the national mortality
register. The study found that the risk of violent death was inversely
related to serum cholesterol level (Vartiainen *et al.* 1994).

3.3.1   What type of study is this and what are the advantages and disadvantages of this design in the study of violent death and serum cholesterol?

3.3.2   What population does the random sample in this study represent?

3.4   *Prima Magazine*, a glossy magazine for women, printed a survey on family life in its January 1999 issue. Thousands of responses were obtained
from the 1.2 million readers, who cover a broad social spectrum. A
random selection of the questionnaires were analysed and the results
presented in the March issue (Prima Magazine 1999, Milne 1999). The
results were all presented as simple percentages of respondents expressing particular views, such as marriage being vital for stable family life.

3.4.1   What biases might there be in this sample of the women of the UK?

3.4.2   What function does random sampling serve here?

ANSWERS

3.3.1 This is a cohort study which starts with the risk factor, serum cholesterol. The sample was identified and serum cholesterol level was measured. The subjects were then followed up and deaths from accident, poisoning or violence were recorded. The study then investigated whether the level of serum cholesterol was related to the risk of death. The main advantage is that the study is prospective. It would be difficult to obtain serum cholesterol after death. The disadvantage is that the study takes a long time to reach its conclusions. It also requires a relatively large sample to provide enough deaths to study and is expensive (*Intro* §3.7).

3.3.2 The sample was drawn from all people born between 1913 and 1947 and living in North Karalla, Finland. Since it is a random sample, it is representative of these individuals. The results of the study may or may not be generalized to other cohorts living in the same area but born at different times and similarly may or may not be generalized to individuals from other places. The generalizability of the findings to another population will depend on how similar the other population is to the Finnish one with respect to characteristics related to serum cholesterol and violent death (*Intro* §3.5).

3.4.1 First, the magazine may have a broad readership, but it will not be a representative sample of women in the UK. It might exclude the very poor and the illiterate, for example. We are not told what proportion of the readership replied, only that it was 'thousands' out of 1.2 million, but it can be only a very small fraction. These may be women who have a particular interest in the topics covered in the questionnaire, for example, or have some special point of view which they wish to communicate. These unknown biases will be present in the thousands of questionnaires returned, and so will be equally present in the random sample drawn for analysis (*Intro* §3.3).

3.4.2 The random sample will be representative of the questionnaires returned. By analysing only a random sample of the questionnaires, the magazine was able to quickly summarize and present the views of thousands of respondents. It would be very unusual for a medical research survey to be published within a year of questionnaires being sent out. This was done within 2 months (*Intro* §3.4).

QUESTIONS

3.5   One hundred and forty-one babies who developed cerebral palsy were compared to a group of babies made up from the two babies immediately after each cerebral palsy baby in the hospital delivery book. Hospital notes were reviewed by a researcher who was blind to the baby's outcome. Failure to respond to signs of fetal distress was noted in 25.8% of the cerebral palsy babies and in 7.1% of the delivery book babies (Gaffney *et al.* 1994).

3.5.1   What kind of study design is this and what are the advantages and disadvantages of this design?

3.5.2   What is meant by blind in this study and why was it done?

3.6   Eighty-seven patients with bronchioalveolar cancer, a rare condition, were compared to 286 non-cancer patients and 297 patients with other types of cancer, matched by age, sex, and race. They were interviewed about their history of cigarette smoking. A strong relationship was observed between smoking and bronchioalveolar cancer (Morabia and Wynder 1992).

What kind of study is this and what are the advantages and disadvantages of this design here?

3.7   In a prospective study of serum sialic acid concentration and cardiovascular mortality, 54 385 men and women aged 40–74 were followed over 20 years. There were 4 420 deaths due to cardiovascular disease and 4 526 non-cardiovascular deaths. The quartiles of sialic acid concentration were used to divide the men into four equal groups. The overall risk of death in the group with the highest fourth of sialic acid concentration was 2.38 times that in the lowest fourth. This association was stronger for cardiovascular deaths than for non-cardiovascular deaths (Lindberg *et al.* 1991).

What kind of study is this and what are the advantages and disadvantages?

3.8   In a study of blood pressure during pregnancy and fetal growth, 209 healthy women having their first baby had 24-hour blood pressure readings taken in early-, mid-, and late-pregnancy. The size of the baby was recorded at birth. The study found that raised blood pressure at 28 weeks gestation was associated with lower mean birthweight and lower ponderal index (Churchill and Beevers 1997).

What kind of study is this and why is this approach suited to the study of the outcome of pregnancy?

ANSWERS

3.5.1   This is a case–control study where the cases are babies with cerebral palsy and the controls are babies born in the same unit at about the same time but without cerebral palsy. The study looks back in time for differences between the cerebral palsy babies and the controls to investigate factors related to the condition. The advantages of the design are that as we start with the cases, the study is relatively quick to do and requires a smaller total sample size than a cohort study investigating the same question, as cerebral palsy is rare. Case–control studies often have the disadvantages that the information is collected retrospectively and may be affected by the condition, and that the choice of control group affects the comparisons that are made. None of these appear to apply to this study (*Intro* §3.8).

3.5.2   Blind means that the researcher was unaware of which babies were cases and controls when he/she reviewed the hospital notes. If the researcher did know, it might (unconsciously or consciously) affect how carefully the notes were searched or how information in the notes was interpreted according to prior beliefs or expectations (*Intro* §2.9).

3.6   This is a case–control study which is used to study the possible causes of bronchioalveolar cancer. The cases are patients with bronchioalveolar cancer, the controls are patients with other cancers or no cancer. The advantages are that we need a relatively small sample, compared with a cohort study which would have to be enormous to collect enough cases as the cancer is rare. The disadvantages are that the choice of the control group may affect results. The inclusion of two separate control groups attempts to allow for this. In addition there may be recall bias associated with smoking history—cases may conceal or exaggerate their habit (*Intro* §3.8).

3.7   This is a cohort study which starts with the risk factor, sialic acid concentration. The study group was followed up over 20 years and deaths and their causes were recorded. The advantage is that the risk factor was ascertained before the event took place, avoiding recall bias and allowing risks to be estimated directly. The disadvantage is that the study takes a long time, is expensive and that subjects may be lost to follow-up (*Intro* §3.7).

3.8   This is a cohort study where the women's blood pressure was monitored during pregnancy and then compared with the birthweight of the baby. Since the length of pregnancy is relatively short, about 40 weeks, the women do not need to be monitored for too long. In addition, women are routinely monitored during pregnancy and so loss to follow-up is minimized. Thus, the study permits relationships between pregnancy factors and birthweight to be investigated (*Intro* §3.7).

QUESTIONS

3.9　Forty-five alcoholic patients and 23 non-alcoholic research or laboratory staff were studied (Sherman *et al.* 1993). A two allele polymorphism was identified and subjects were classified into three genotypes, AA, AB, and BB. The results were:

	Genotype		
	BB	AA	BA
Alcoholic patients	19	7	19
Non-alcoholic subjects	2	18	3

3.9.1　Why is the case–control approach particularly suitable here?

3.9.2　What problems might result from using research or laboratory staff as the control group?

3.10　Infants who died from Sudden Infant Death Syndrome (SIDS or cot death) were compared to a group of live infants, matched for age and birthweight. The temperature in the baby's bedroom and the amount of thermal insulation (clothes and bedding) were measured, to give an estimate of the excess thermal insulation. The study found that the dead children had had more excess thermal insulation than the live children. Infants who died were also more likely than live infants to have been laid to sleep in the prone position (Ponsonby *et al.* 1992).

3.10.1　What are the advantages and disadvantages of this design to study cot deaths?

3.10.2　Why are age and birthweight good variables to match for?

3.11　In a study of the effect of breast feeding on infections in babies, 750 mothers and their infants were observed several times during the first 2 years of the baby's life. Babies breast fed for 13 weeks or more had less gastrointestinal illness that those bottle fed from birth. However, the bottle feeding mothers and breast feeding mothers differed. For example, 85% of bottle feeders had left school at age 16 or less, compared to 36% of breast feeders. The statistical analysis adjusted for some of these differences. All women lived in Dundee and were in a stable relationship. All babies who were born early, had low birth weight or required special care were excluded (Howie *et al.* 1990).

3.11.1　Can we conclude that bottle feeding causes infection?

3.11.2　Why was it a good idea to exclude babies who were born early, had low birthweight or required special care?

3.11.3　What factors should we take into account in applying this result to babies in general?

ANSWERS

3.9.1   The design is suitable because we can identify alcoholics fairly readily from those attending for treatment. There is no recall problem because genotype cannot change over time. We cannot identify genotype without obtaining blood and carrying out a test. A case–control design minimizes the number of tests needed (*Intro* §3.8).

3.9.2   The problem is that cases and controls are not drawn from the same population and so might not be comparable. If this gene were related to success in higher education, for example, it would affect the chance of being in the control group rather than the case group (*Intro* §3.8).

3.10.1 This is a case–control study in which the cases are babies who died, the controls are babies who did not die. SIDS is a rare event and so this design will give a quicker result than a cohort study and will require a smaller sample size. Since thermal insulation was measured directly rather than being recalled, there is no recall bias, but there is potential for considerable assessment bias. There may be recall bias in reporting sleeping position and temperature may have changed. The choice of control group may also affect the results (*Intro* §3.8).

3.10.2 Both the age and birthweight of the baby are related to the amount of clothing which the baby wears and the way in which the baby is laid to sleep and also to the risk of cot death. Matching for these variables thus allows a better assessment of the effect of excess clothes and bedding (*Intro* §3.8).

3.11.1 This is an observational study not a randomized trial. Breast and bottle feeders are self-selected and differ in many ways, e.g. education. The analysis was only adjusted for some of these, there may be others we do not know about. All we can say is that bottle feeding and infection are associated, not that one causes the other.

3.11.2 These babies condition might influence the decision about feeding method, making them less likely to be breast fed. Their condition might also increase their risk of infection, because their immune system is less developed, for example. Thus including them might produce a spurious relationship between feeding method and infections.

3.11.3 These results apply to women living in Dundee in stable relationships with normal term births. It seems unlikely that there would be a difference in Dundee and not elsewhere, or in women with stable relationships but not in others. The magnitude of the relationship might not be the same. The circumstances of pre-term, small, and special care births are so different that we cannot extend the results to them.

QUESTIONS

3.12   A group of 918 women with breast cancer diagnosed before age 55 were interviewed about their past use of oral contraceptives. For each woman, a woman without cancer, of the same age and living in the same area, was chosen at random from a population register and interviewed also. The study showed a positive relationship between the duration of oral contraception use and breast cancer (Rookus and van Leeuwen 1994).

     What are the advantages and disadvantages of this design to study contraceptive use and early breast cancer?

3.13   Doctors have observed that hand injuries occurring in the home form a substantial proportion of hand injuries seen at A&E departments and further that an increasing number of these injuries are caused by the person trying to separate packed frozen food. To investigate this they therefore reviewed the case notes of patients at four hospitals plus the Department of Trade's home accident surveillance system database for similar injuries. Between 1992 and 1995, cases were identified by alerted surgeons and by reviewing the notes of patients with knife wounds, supplemented where necessary by telephone interview with the patient. The researchers commented that they probably missed some cases because records do not always specify how an injury has occurred (Jigjinni 1997).

     Twenty-seven hospital patients were identified plus 32 patients from the database. All injuries were to the non-dominant hand with 11 injuries to the palm and 16 to the fingers. The majority of injuries were treated by hand surgeons with only six patients having skin lacerations alone. In each group of patients, beefburgers were the food most commonly responsible for the accidents, although chops, sausages, crumpets and pastry also featured in both groups.

3.13.1   What is the purpose of the study and what type of study is it?

3.13.2   What were the limitations of the study?

3.13.3   The authors concluded that hand injury is common and preventable. What further information would be useful in judging the scale of the problem?

ANSWERS

3.12   This is a case–control study where the cases are women with breast cancer and the controls are women of the same age in the same area who do not have breast cancer. The advantages are that an answer will be obtained more quickly and with a smaller sample than a cohort study. The disadvantages are firstly selection bias whereby women who are taking oral contraception may be in more frequent contact with health services and so be more likely to be screened for breast cancer. Also there may be recall bias, since recall of contraceptive use may be influenced by the disease (*Intro* §3.8).

3.13.1 The study was set up to investigate patients who had injured their hands while separating frozen food and to demonstrate that this is a important problem, although this was not explicitly stated. The study design was a case-series because it was a descriptive study of a group of patients with a common condition (hand injury) (*Intro* §3.5).

3.13.2 The authors admit that they may have missed some cases and so the condition may be more frequent than the data suggest (*Intro* §3.5).

3.13.3 Twenty-seven hospital cases over 3 years is about two cases per hospital per year which does not appear to be very common. No denominators were give to show what rates of injury there were (*Intro* §3.5).

QUESTIONS

3.14 A paper about new variant Creutzfeldt–Jakob disease (nvCJD) and bovine pituitary growth hormone discussed a French patient who died of nvCJD in January 1996 following an illness of 23 months. It was noted that in the UK there had been only one patient in whom clinical onset occurred earlier than in this French man. It was reported that this patient was a devoted body-builder. Although at the time human growth hormone was not used in France to increase muscle strength, a bovine form of the drug was sometimes prescribed for 'tissue repairs'. This drug was banned in July 1992. It was suggested that the French case of nvCJD diagnosed in February 1994 is compatible with an inoculation having occurred during the late 1980s (Verdrager 1998).

What type of study is this, and what the strengths and limitations of such a design?

3.15 A cross-sectional study investigated the association between raised body temperature and acute mountain sickness in 60 climbers in Switzerland. The climbers were examined at low altitude (490 m above sea level), 2–6 hours after arrival at a mountain hut at 4 559 m and each morning during the next 3 days. Each day, symptoms and signs of acute mountain sickness were assessed and climbers were classified as healthy, as having mild acute mountain sickness or as having severe acute mountain illness. Climbers were also classified as having or not having high altitude cerebral or pulmonary oedema according to symptoms and chest radiography. Body temperature and blood gases were also measured. Fifteen climbers who were found to have cerebral or pulmonary oedema were evacuated by helicopter (Maggiorini *et al.* 1997).

The study showed a strong relation between body temperature, hypoxaemia and the severity of acute mountain sickness on the same day. The researchers concluded that a rise in temperature after rapid ascent to high altitude is a sign of acute mountain sickness and is associated with the severity of hypoxaemia.

3.15.1 Why is this a cross-sectional study?

3.15.2 The study was approved by the ethics committee of the University Hospital Zurich. Do you think that this study was ethical?

ANSWERS

3.14   This is a clinical case study which describes and discusses in detail the medical condition of one patient. This design is useful in reporting on rare conditions (such as nvCJD, here) and allows fuller clinical details to be given than is possible in a multi-patient study. They can be used as here, to suggest a causal mechanism for the condition or in other cases to draw clinicians' attention to a rare event. The limitations are that we cannot necessarily generalize from one patient to all patients with the same condition and that any hypotheses raised need to be tested in other studies with several patients (*Intro* §3.5).

3.15.1   The study is cross-sectional because it looks at the relationship between variables measured at the same time, i.e. it investigated severity of mountain sickness score and temperature in the 60 climbers at the same time.

3.15.2   This was a very unusual study because they deliberately set out to make the subjects ill. Presumably the climbers had experience of altitude and knew what they were letting themselves in for, though no mention is made of how consent was obtained. One-quarter of the climbers had to be evacuated by helicopter. Thus, the ethics of this study would seem to be debateable.

QUESTIONS

3.16   Questionnaires were sent to 60 000 readers of a consumer magazine, asking about illness experienced in connection with holidays in 1997–8 (*Holiday Which?* 1999). The analysis presented was based on more than 23 500 questionnaires. The response rate was about 50%, which is quite good for a postal survey.

Overall, 12% of respondents reported illness, an increase from the 10% reported in a similar survey the previous year. The greatest proportion was among the 72 visitors to Mexico (58%), followed by the Dominican Republic, Egypt, and India, and so on down to the smallest proportion among the 129 visitors to Belgium (5%), with Croatia, UK, and Hong Kong in the places immediately above (*Holiday Which?* 1999).

❗ 3.16.1   What effect might the incomplete response have on the proportions reported to have experienced illness?

❗ 3.16.2   What effect might the incomplete response have on the relative ordering of the countries?

❗ 3.16.3   What effect might the incomplete response have on the difference between the two surveys?

❗ 3.16.4   Apart from differences between countries in food, in hygiene, etc., could any other factor explain some of the variation in reported illness between them?

❗ 3.16.5   The report says that 'Easily the worst country for illness was Mexico ...where more people fell ill than not. The proportion of people succumbing to sickness in Mexico has more than doubled, from 27 per cent in our last survey to 58 per cent this time.' How reliable do you think this change might be?

3.17   In a study of suicide and social factors, data were analysed for the 633 parliamentary constituencies of Great Britain. For each constituency, suicide rates were calculated for men and women in several age groups. For each constituency, the Townsend socio-economic deprivation score was calculated using census data on unemployment, car ownership, overcrowded housing, and housing tenure. Congdon's social fragmentation (anomie) index was derived from census data on private renting, single person households, unmarried persons, and mobility in the previous year. Mean voter abstention rates were calculated from four general elections. Higher voter abstention, social fragmentation, and Townsend scores were associated with higher suicide rates in all age and sex groups. The association was greatest for social fragmentation (Whitley *et al.* 1999).

➕ 3.17.1   What kind of study is this?

3.17.2   Can we conclude that social fragmentation causes suicide?

ANSWERS

3.16.1 It may be that people who were sent the questionnaire would be more likely to reply if they had had problems with their holiday than if they had not. (This is our personal experience of being in the sample for this survey on two occasions.) Thus, there may be an upward bias in the proportions who were ill (*Intro* §3.4).

3.16.2 The bias may be the same for all countries. It is less plausible that people who became ill in Hong Kong were less likely to respond than people who became ill in Egypt. The response rate may not affect the order (*Intro* §3.5).

3.16.3 The bias should be the same in the two surveys, which used the same methodology. Thus the increase in illness is fairly reliable. This may reflect a worldwide increase in infection, or, more plausibly, an increase in the number of people taking holidays in less developed countries.

3.16.4 The people who holiday in Mexico and India may be more adventurous and hence more likely to take risks in general than those who holiday in the UK and Belgium. This is not the only explanation, however, as Croatia and Hong Kong show.

3.16.5 Mexico is picked out because it is the largest. It is very likely that it will have increased from the previous survey to become so. Thus it may be the selection of Mexico which highlights a chance difference, rather than a genuine increase of this magnitude. This phenomenon, where the top of a league table in 1 year is lower down in other years, is an example of regression towards the mean and is caused by random variation (*Intro* §11.4).

3.17.1 This is an ecological study, which relates the incidence of disease (suicide) to the characteristics of the areas where people live (*Intro3* §3.10).

3.17.2 We cannot conclude that social fragmentation causes suicide. We should always be cautious about concluding from an observational study that one variable causes another. Furthermore, as the authors of this study point out: 'It is important to recognize the limitations of ecological studies. Although socially fragmented areas have higher suicide rates, the people who commit suicide may not share the characteristics of the populations from which they are drawn. Moreover, the direction of the association is unclear, and it may be that people at high risk of suicide choose to live in socially fragmented areas or that these areas contain more hostels for mentally ill people.' (Whitley *et al.* 1999). To conclude that there was a relationship at the level of the individual would be an example of the ecological fallacy (*Intro3* §3.10).

4
Summarizing data

This chapter covers frequency, histograms, means and standard deviations.

A variable has different values for different members of the population, e.g. whether people smoke, how many children they have, their height. Qualitative variables have no numerical value, e.g. whether people smoke. Quantitative variables have numerical value and may be discrete, with only a few possible values, e.g. how many children, or continuous, being able to take any value within a range, e.g. height. A set of observations of a variable form a distribution.

A frequency is the number of times a particular value occurs. A frequency distribution is the set of frequencies for all possible values. For continuous variables we divide the scale into class intervals and find the frequency for each interval. A frequency distribution may be graphed as a histogram, a frequency polygon, a box and whisker plot, or a stem and leaf plot.

A quantile divides a frequency distribution in a given ratio. For example, the median, the value so that half the observations are greater than it and half are less, splits the distribution into two equal parts. The three quartiles divide the ordered data into four equal parts, called fourths. The first quartile has 25% of the observations below it, the second (the median) has 50% below it, and the third quartile has 75% of observations below it.

The mean is the arithmetic average of the observations. The geometric mean is found by multiplying all n observations and taking the nth root. In a symmetrical distribution, the mean and median are approximately equal, in a positively skew distribution the mean is the larger.

The range is a measure of variation, the difference between the largest and smallest observations, sometimes quoted as the smallest to the largest. It may vary a lot from sample to sample, since it does not use all the information, and it depends on the sample size.

The variance is a measure of variation, the average squared difference from the mean. It is in squared units. For a sample, it is estimated by the sum of squares about the mean divided by the degrees of freedom (the sample size minus one). The standard deviation is the square root of the variance. It is in the same units as the variable. For the majority of observations (about 2/3) the difference between observation and mean will be less than one standard deviation and nearly all these differences (about 95%) will be less than two standard deviations.

QUESTIONS

4.1   In a study of blood pressure in one town, the distribution of diastolic
blood pressure among men was shown as follows (Hawthorne *et al.*
1974):

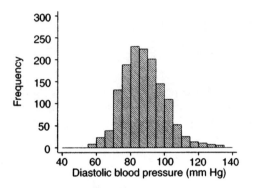

4.1.1   What kind of diagram is this?

4.1.2   How would you describe the shape of the distribution?

4.1.3   The class intervals are 5 mm Hg wide. In what interval would a diastolic
blood pressure of 70 be put in?

4.2   In a review article on myelodysplastic syndromes (Oscier 1997), the age
distribution of patients presenting in one town was shown as follows:

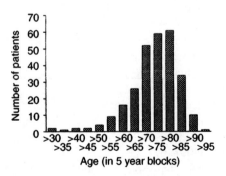

4.2.1   What is the shape of the distribution?

4.2.2   Could the presentation of the figure be improved?

ANSWERS

4.1.1   We would call this a histogram (*Intro* §4.3).

4.1.2   The distribution has a slight positive skew or is skew to the right, the
         longer tail being on the right (*Intro* §4.4).

4.1.3   The convention is to include the lower limit in the interval, thus the
         interval which starts at 65 and finishes at 70 does not actually include
         70, which is put into the interval 70–75 (*Intro* §4.2).

4.2.1   The long tail is on the left, so the distribution is skew to the left or
         negatively skew (*Intro* §4.4).

4.2.2   Since age is continuous, there is no need to put gaps between the ver-
         tical bars. These gaps suggest that there are gaps in the distribution,
         which there are not. The distribution could be shown as a conventional
         histogram:

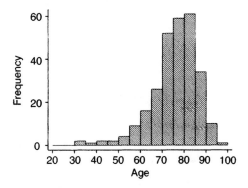

QUESTIONS

4.3   The general health questionnaire (GHQ) is a measure of psychological
        morbidity. It consists of a series of 12 questions each with four possible
        answers, usually of the form 'not at all', 'same as usual', 'more than
        usual', and 'much more than usual'. These can be scored 0, 1, 2, or 3
        and the scores added to give a total GHQ score between 0 and 36. Paw-
        likowska *et al.* (1994) obtained GHQ scores from 15 283 subjects drawn
        from GP lists. They presented a graph similar to this:

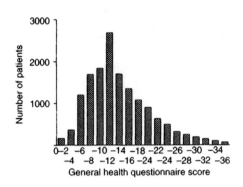

4.3.1   What is the shape of this frequency distribution?

4.3.2   What is unusual about the class intervals?

❗ 4.3.3   What problems are there in drawing a histogram for these data and how
        could they be resolved?

4.3.4   The authors quote the mean GHQ scores for men and women as 24.7
        and 26.2, respectively. Is this plausible?

4.4   Infants who died from sudden infant death syndrome (SIDS or cot death)
        were compared to a group of live infants, matched for age and birth-
        weight. The temperature in the baby's bedroom and the amount of
        thermal insulation (clothes and bedding) were measured, to give an
        estimate of the excess thermal insulation. The dead children had had
        more excess thermal insulation (mean 2.3 togs, standard deviation 3.4
        togs) than the live children (mean 0.6 togs, standard deviation 2.3 togs)
        (Ponsonby *et al.* 1992).

4.4.1   What is meant by mean and standard deviation?

❗ 4.4.2   What do they tell us here about the shape of the distribution?

ANSWERS

4.3.1   The tail on the right is the longer, so the distribution is skew to the right or positively skew (*Intro* §4.4).

4.3.2   The first class interval is bigger than the rest, covering three possible values of the GHQ score, 0, 1, and 2. All the others cover only two possible values, –4 covers 3 and 4, for example. The statistical convention is for the interval to include the lower limit, not the upper limit. It would therefore be more usual for the intervals to be 0–1, 2–, 4–, etc. (*Intro* §4.2).

4.3.3   The score is discrete, taking only integer values. It is limited at 0 and 36 and both limits are achieved in this data set. Since the data set is so large it would be possible to give each integer between 0 and 36 its own class interval, giving 37 bars altogether.

4.3.4   As all respondents are either men or women, the mean for the whole sample must be somewhere between 24.7 and 26.2, about 25.6. Judging from the graph, the mean is about 14.0. For more on this obvious discrepancy, see Bland (2000a), Chalder and Wessely (2000), and on the World Wide Web http://www.bmj.com/cgi/eletters/320/7233/515/a#EL1.

4.4.1   The mean or average is the sum of all the observations divided by the number of observations and gives a measure of the centrality of the data. The standard deviation is a measure of the scatter of the data about the mean value and is measured in the same units as the data itself. It is the square root of the variance where the variance of the sample is given by the sum of the squared deviations from the mean divided by the total sample size minus one (*Intro* §4.6, 4.8).

4.4.2   If the data were symmetrically distributed, we would expect about 2.5% of the observations to be less than the mean minus 2 standard deviations. For a variable which can only take positive values, we can deduce positive skewness where the standard deviation is bigger than half the mean. However, here the variable is excess insulation where negative values are possible and so we cannot deduce the shape of the distribution from these values.

QUESTIONS

4.5   Cotinine is an indicator of exposure to cigarette smoke. In a study of maternal cotinine level during pregnancy and subsequent birthweight, women who did not themselves smoke during pregnancy were grouped by whether there was a cigarette smoker in the home. The following figure was presented:

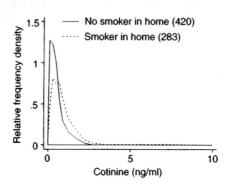

4.5.1   What kind of figure is this?

4.5.2   How would you describe the shape of these distributions and what does the figure tell us about cotinine and smoking in the home?

4.5.3   Why is relative frequency density shown rather than frequency?

The mothers were divided into five equal groups according to the level of cotinine in their blood. The following data were presented:

Cotinine (ng/ml)	0–0.180	0.181–0.291	0.292–0.480	0.481–0.795	0.796+
Number of women	169	159	162	164	164
Mean birth-weight (g)	3 445	3 453	3 411	3 365	3 372

The authors reported that the difference in mean birthweight between non-smokers in the lower and upper quintiles of cotinine was 0.2% (95% confidence interval −2.4% to 2.8%) (Peacock *et al.* 1998).

4.5.4   What are the quintiles? Why is the use of the term here incorrect? What term would be better?

4.6   The following statement appeared in a letter from a British Labour Party spin-doctor in a national newspaper: 'The average income of the middle quartile of earners (40–60% of the population) is £326 a week ...' (The Guardian 1999).

4.6.1   What is wrong with this statement?

4.6.2   What is the more usual name for the 'middle quartile'?

ANSWERS

4.5.1   The graph shows two frequency polygons (*Intro* §4.3).

4.5.2   The distributions are positively skew. Although there is a lot of overlap, the women with smokers in the home appear to have higher cotinine levels (*Intro* §4.4).

4.5.3   The numbers in the two groups are different, so using relative frequency, the proportion of observations in the interval or cell, makes the two shapes easier to compare than using the frequencies would. Frequency density, the number of observations per unit of cotinine, makes it possible to use intervals of different widths, as in this figure (*Intro* §4.2, 4.4).

4.5.4   The quintiles are the values such that one-fifth of the observations are below the first quintile, two-fifths are below the second quintile, etc. There are four of them. In this study the quintiles are the cut-off values between the five equal-sized groups: 0.180 5, 0.291 5, 0.480 5 and 0.795 5. The term is often incorrectly used for the five equal-sized groups which splitting the observations at the quintile produces. A better term would be 'fifths'. The authors of this paper included four statisticians, of whom Bland and Peacock were two! They also meant lowest and highest, not lower and upper (*Intro* §4.5).

4.6.1   The three quartiles are the values which divide the distribution into four equal parts. They are points, not groups of people. They therefore do not have averages. The word is sometimes incorrectly used to mean one of the four groups into which the three quartiles divide the population, more correctly called 'fourths'. In this sense there is no 'middle quartile' because there are four of them and each fourth contains 25% of the population (*Intro* §4.5). (The newspaper in question is notorious for misprints, so this may not be quite what the author wrote.)

4.6.2   The middle quartile is the median (*Intro* §4.5).

QUESTIONS

4.7   In a study of the use of alternative medicines, households were randomly selected from Adelaide and country centres in South Australia.
Three thousand and four people were interviewed; 48.5% of respondents
used at least one non-prescribed alternative medicine. The estimated
monthly cost for users of alternative medicines ranged from $AU1 to
$AU500, median $AU10 (MacLennan *et al.* 1996).

4.7.1   What is meant by 'ranged from $AU1 to $AU500, median $AU10' and
what does this tell us about the shape of the distribution of expenditure?

4.7.2   If all respondents were included in the distribution of monthly cost,
what would the median be?

4.8   In a study of patients admitted to an otolaryngology ward, 140 patients
with nose-bleeds were compared to 113 controls with other conditions.
Patients were interviewed about their alcohol consumption (McGarry
et al. 1994). The results for the number of units of alcohol consumed
per week were:

	Nose-bleed patients ($n = 140$)	Other patients ($n = 113$)
Median	10.0	2.0
Interquartile range	0–50	0–10

One unit of alcohol is half-a-pint beer, a glass of wine, or a pub measure of spirits.

4.8.1   What is meant by 'median' and 'interquartile range'? Why are they
used here?

4.8.2   What is the shape of the distribution of alcohol consumption?

4.9   To investigate the effect of Phase 3 of the NHS and Community Care Act
on hospital practice, 2 groups of patients were compared: 100 discharged
before the introduction of the act and 100 discharged after.

The 100 patients before the act accounted for 8 875 patient bed days
(median 63 days per patient) and the 100 patients after the act
accounted for 7 131 patient bed days (median 35 days per patient) (Ajayi
et al. 1995).

❗ 4.9.1   The mean numbers of days per patient were 88.75 and 71.31, respectively. Why might the median numbers of days per patient be less than
the means here?

❗ 4.9.2   Why did they quote the medians rather than the means?

ANSWERS

4.7.1   Ranged from $AU1 to $AU500 means that the smallest observation was $AU1 and the largest was $AU500. The median is the expenditure so that half the expenditures are greater than it and half are less. Since the number of subjects is even, it is the average of the two central values. As the median is close to the minimum, the distribution is probably highly skew to the right (*Intro* §4.5, 4.7).

4.7.2   Zero, since more than half the respondents did not use alternative medicines.

4.8.1   The median is the central point in a set of observations when they are ordered from the smallest to the largest. Hence half of the observations lie above the median and half lie below it. Because it is the central point in the ordered data, it is not affected by extreme values and so may be a better descriptive summary measure for skewed data such as alcohol consumption.

The lower and upper quartiles are the points such that a quarter of the observations lie below the lower quartile and a quarter lie above the upper quartile. The interval between the lower and upper quartile is known as the interquartile range. Hence the interquartile range gives a range of values which includes half of the observations. It, too, is unaffected by the most extreme observations.

In this example we can see that median alcohol consumption is higher in nose-bleed patients than in controls. The interquartile ranges both start at zero, showing that at least one quarter of each group were non-drinkers. However, the third quartile for nose-bleed patients (50 units) was considerably higher than for controls (10 units) showing that the heaviest drinkers in the nose-bleed patients were drinking more than the heaviest drinkers in the control group. Thus, the nose-bleed patients had greater variability in alcohol consumption than other patients (*Intro* §4.5, 4.7).

4.8.2   The medians are much closer to the first quartiles than to the third quartiles. The distribution of alcohol consumption is therefore positively skew for both groups (*Intro* §4.4).

4.9.1   The distribution of the number of days in hospital is likely to be positively skewed because a few patients stay for a very long time. For positively skewed data, the few high values at the upper end of the range will have a disproportionate effect on the mean, increasing its value. Hence the median will be less than the mean for such data (*Intro* §4.5, 4.6).

4.9.2   In this situation the median is a better measure of the centre of the distribution since it is less affected by extreme values (*Intro* §4.5).

QUESTIONS

4.10   The following extract is from *Hansard*, 29 November 1991, quoted in *Royal Statistical Society News and Notes*, 1992 Vol. 18(7), p. 12). The idea which Members of Parliament are discussing is that a minimum wage would be defined as a fixed proportion of the median wage.

Mr. Arbuthnot: ...suggestion of a minimum wage is in itself rather obscure and bizarre. As I understand it, it is tied to the average and would therefore not only be relatively high at £3.40, but would increase as the average wage itself increased. With each increase in the average rate of pay, the minimum wage itself would have to go up and it would be forever chasing its own tail.

Mr. Tony Lloyd: Perhaps I can help the Hon. Gentleman. It will be tied to the median, which is not the same as the average. It is simply the mid-point on the range and would not be affected by changes in the minimum wage.

Mr. Arbuthnot: From what I understand, even an amount tied to the median would be affected because if the lowest wage were increased to £3.40 per hour, the median would have to rise.

Mr. Tony Lloyd: I shall put the matter in simple terms. The median, the mid-point in a series of numbers such as 2, 2, 5, 6, and 7, is defined as being the difference between 2 and 7, which is 3.5. If we alter the figures 2 and 2 to 3.5, the middle figure of 5 would remain unaltered because it is independent of the bottom figures.

Mr. Arbuthnot: I do not understand the Hon. Gentleman's mathematics and I slightly doubt whether he does.

Mr. Matthew Carrington: I am extremely confused. I studied mathematics for some years at school and I have not totally forgotten all of them. The median is not the mid-point between the first number and the last. It is where the largest number of items in a sample comes to, whereas the average is obviously the sample multiplied by the number of items. The Hon. Member for Stretford (Mr. Lloyd) is obviously extremely confused. The median has a precise mathematical definition which is absolutely right, and my Hon. Friend is correct in saying that the median is bound to alter if the number at the bottom of the scale is changed. That will alter the average as well in a different way, but it is bound to alter the median. Perhaps the Hon. Member for Stretford wishes to define median in a non-mathematical sense.

Mr. Arbuthnot: I am extremely grateful to my Hon. Friend for sorting out at least the Hon. Gentleman's mathematics with obvious skill and knowledge.

4.10.1   Which Honourable Member is correct, if any, and why?

ANSWERS

4.10.1   Mr. Lloyd is correct that the mean is not the same as the median but
         his definition of the median is wrong. It is the middle number when the
         numbers are arranged in ascending order and not the difference between
         the minimum and maximum values. So using his first example (2, 2,
         5, 6, 7), the median here would be 5 and not 3.5 as asserted. He is
         correct that altering the extreme values will not change the median but
         his argument is confused.

         Mr Carrington is correct that the median is not the mid-point between
         the first number and the last but is wrong in his definition. His definition
         appears to be referring to the mode of a distribution, i.e. the category
         which has the highest frequency, although his explanation is not very
         clear. His definition of the average is wrong (the sample multiplied by
         the number of items). He is wrong in stating that the median will change
         if the number at the bottom of the scale changes. This will not change
         the median but will alter the mean (*Intro* §4.5).

QUESTIONS

❗ 4.10.2   What would be the effect on the skewness of the earnings distribution if the minimum wage were made a fixed proportion of the median, assuming that this figure was then higher than the current wage of some members of the population?

4.11   In a study of the relationship between ethnic group of applicants for medical school and rating of application forms, forms were given to assessors either open as sent or with the name and other ethnic group cues obliterated, so that assessment was blind. The forms were scored out of 20 for suitability for interview, a different assessor rating the masked and open forms for the same applicant. Ethnic group was classified (by different observers) from the form as either European, unidentified ethnic minority, or identified ethnic minority (Lumb and Vail 2000). The following figure was presented (thanks to Andy Vail for letting us have the data):

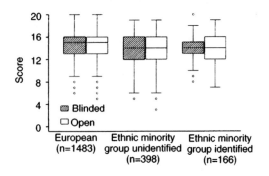

➕ 4.11.1   What kind of graph is this?

➕ 4.11.2   In the plot, what do the five horizontal lines for each group represent?

➕ 4.11.3   What does the graph tell us about the shapes of the distributions?

➕ 4.11.4   What can we conclude from this figure?

➕ 4.11.5   Why are there a number of observations shown as isolated points?

❗➕ 4.11.6   How could the data be plotted so as to take the paired structure into account?

❗➕ 4.11.7   What might such a plot obscure and what might it reveal?

ANSWERS

4.10.2   The distribution would become more positively skew. The smallest wages would be increased and the short, left-hand tail of the distribution would be made even shorter (*Intro* §4.4).

4.11.1   This is a box and whisker plot (*Intro* §4.3).

4.11.2   The middle line is the median, the lines at the bottom and top of the box are the first and third quartiles, i.e. there are 25% of the observations below the box and 25% above it. The bottom and top lines represent the minimum and maximum observations (*Intro* §4.3).

4.11.3   The shapes of the distributions appear to be fairly symmetrical, though there might be a slight negative skewness.

4.11.4   We can conclude that distribution of scores is virtually identical whether the forms are open or blinded, and in particular that the median scores are the same.

4.11.5   These points are extreme, quite a long way from the rest of the data. They have been separated from the rest of the data. The usual convention is that points are regarded as 'outside' if they are further than 1.5 times the interquartile range from the quartile, i.e. from the edge of the box. Such points are sometimes shown separately from the whiskers, as here, sometimes included within the whisker (*Intro* §4.3).

4.11.6   The graph shown does not make any connection between the paired scores on the blinded and open forms. One possibility would be to plot the differences between masked and open, like this:

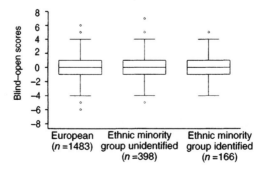

Several other approaches could be used, but there are too many points for scatter diagrams.

4.11.7   It is very clear that median difference in score is zero. The close similarity between the whole distribution for the blinded and open assessments is obscured. What is brought out is the considerable variation in the scores given to the same form by different assessors.

QUESTIONS

4.12   In a study of muscle training in patients with rheumatoid arthritis, patients were randomized to receive either a standardized exercise regime or normal care (McKeeken *et al.* 1999). Measurements were made before and after 6 weeks' treatment. The observer was blind to the treatment. The following information was given about the patients in the study:

Characteristic	Exercise group	Control group
Number	17	18
Females (males)	15 (2)	14 (4)
Age (mean ± SD) (years)	51.4 (±11.1)	49.7 (±15.3)
Body weight (mean ± SD) (kg)	71.0 (±23.4)	69.4 (±17.9)
Height (mean ± SD) (m)	1.63 (±0.6)	1.66 (±0.8)

4.12.1   What does 'SD' stand for and what does it mean?

4.12.2   There are two obvious misprints in this table. What are they?

Several outcome variables were measured before and after treatment. Peak speed is the peak angular velocity of the knee movement in rising from a sitting position, measured in degrees per second. TUG is the time to get up and go from a sitting position, in seconds. PVAS is pain measured on a visual analogue scale, where patients are given a 10 cm line, marked 'no pain at all' at one end and 'worst pain you can imagine' at the other. The patient marks the point which they think best represents the pain. The health assessment questionnaire (HAQ) is a scale of limitations on activity, high scores being more limited. The results for these tests, given as mean (±SD), were:

Measure	Control group		Experimental group	
	Pre-treat	Post-treat	Pre-treat	Post-treat
Peak speed $(\deg/s^{-1})$	125.2 (±33.9)	121.6 (±27.7)	132.0 (±40.6)	154.0 (±45.8)
TUG (s)	12.6 (±1.5)	12.2 (±1.3)	11.7 (±1.9)	10.4 (±1.8)
PVAS (mm)	4.1 (±2.4)	3.9 (±2.4)	4.3 (±2.2)	2.4 (±2.1)
HAQ	0.7 (±0.4)	0.8 (±0.3)	1.0 (±0.6)	0.7 (±0.6)

4.12.3   In this table, there are two obvious misprints in the units in which variables are measured. What are they?

4.12.4   Which of the outcome variables must have a skew distribution, from the information in the table alone?

4.12.5   Does the '±' symbol contribute anything?

ANSWERS

4.12.1 'SD' stands for standard deviation. This is a measure of the variability or spread of the data. Approximately 95% of the observations will lie between the mean plus or minus 2 standard deviations (*Intro* §4.8).

4.12.2 The standard deviations for height cannot be correct. These would imply that some heights could be below the mean minus 2SD = 1.63 − 2 × 0.6 = 0.43 m, or above the mean plus 2SD = 1.63 + 2 × 0.6 = 2.83 m, clearly impossible. In fact the standard deviations were 0.06 m and 0.08 m (McKeeken, personal communication).

4.12.3 The units for peak speed should be (deg/s) or (deg s^{-1}), not (deg/s^{-1}). We think the units for PVAS should be cm, not mm. It is implausible that almost all of the subjects will put their marks in the first 10 mm of the 100 mm line.

4.12.4 PVAS and HAQ must have skew distributions, because the standard deviation is greater than half the mean, which would imply negative values if the distributions were symmetrical.

4.12.5 We think the plus or minus symbol can be rather misleading. We are not actually estimating anything to be mean − SD or mean + SD. Most observations will lie between mean − 2SD and mean + 2SD, for example. We think this symbol is at best redundant. We think a better alternative would be to include a heading showing 'mean (SD)' and give the data as '125.2 (33.9)'.

5
Presenting data

Tables and graphs must convey information clearly and quickly. They should not mislead the reader. They should be clearly titled and labelled. Bar charts and line graphs should show the zero value on the axis if possible. Although graphs can convey a lot of information quickly, they can also be very misleading.

Sometimes graphs use a logarithmic scale. The effect is to compress the scale for high values and stretch the scale for low values. This may make positively skew distributions symmetrical. It makes multiplicative relationships additive and may straighten curved relationships. The values 1 and 10 and 10 and 100 are equal distances apart on a logarithmic scale, because they share the same ratio.

QUESTIONS

5.1   All patients admitted with suspected myocardial infarction in the Nottingham health district during 1989 and 1990 were studied to determine whether women received the same therapeutic interventions as men. The following table was given (Clarke *et al.* 1994).

Time from onset of symptoms to arrival in hospital

Time (hours)	No. (%) of men	No. (%) of women
< 6	2 528 (52)	1 404 (47)
6–12	535 (11)	329 (11)
12–24	340 (7)	209 (7)
> 24	1 459 (30)	1 046 (35)
Total	4 862 (100)	2 988 (100)

5.1.1   What features of this table are clear?

5.1.2   What is ambiguous about the time categories?

5.2   In a study of long-term limiting illness and other dimensions of self-reported health, 6 212 men and women completed the SF36 questionnaire to assess their health. For each of 8 sub-scales of the SF36, mean scores were compared for those reporting long-term limiting illness and those not. A graph similar to the following was presented (Cohen *et al.* 1995).

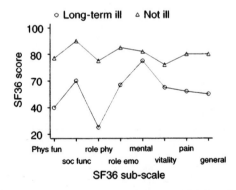

Key: 'phys fun' = physical functioning; 'soc func' = social functioning; 'role phy' = role physical; 'role emo' = role emotional; 'mental' = mental health; 'pain' = bodily pain; 'general' = general health.

5.2.1   What kind of graph is this?

5.2.2   This graph plots mean values on the 8 SF36 sub-scales and joins up points for those with and without long-term illness. What is wrong with this approach? Suggest an alternative graph.

ANSWERS

5.1.1   The table has a clear title, and has headings for all rows and columns. Frequencies and percentages are labelled and the sum of percentages is given at the bottom of the columns to show that percentages are calculated by columns. The units of time are given as 'hours' (*Intro* §5.3).

5.1.2   'Twelve hours' is contained in both the second and third categories. This could be just a typographical error in which case we do not know if those who waited 12 hours are included in the second or third category. Alternatively it could be that those who waited 12 hours are included in both categories and are double-counted.

5.2.1   This is a line graph. Such graphs are usually used to show change in a quantity over time, which is not the case here (*Intro* §5.7).

5.2.2   The 8 SF36 sub-scales are discrete scales, not a continuous scale and so to join them up is meaningless. It suggests some ordering which is not present. A better graph is one where the sub-scales are displayed separately, like the bar graph below. This allows us to compare mean values for those with and without long-term illness on each sub-scale separately.

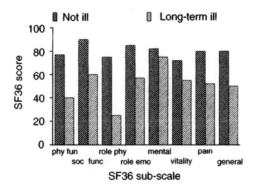

QUESTIONS

5.3   In a study of repetitive strain injury (RSI) and keyboard use, researchers compared skin temperature before and after typing in 10 patients with RSI and in 21 controls without RSI (Sharma *et al.* 1997). The paper included a graph similar to this:

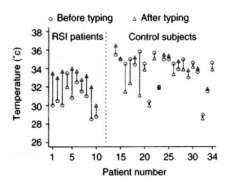

5.3.1   The figure plots the temperature against the patient number. Do you think that patient number is an important variable?

5.3.2   How could the data be plotted more clearly?

5.4   The frequency of arm movements of 25 patients with coronary heart disease (CHD), consecutive attenders at a chest pain clinic, was compared with those of 25 consecutive attenders at a non-cardiac clinic. The study found that the patients with CHD made more arm movements than the controls (Rennie 1997). A graph similar to this was given:

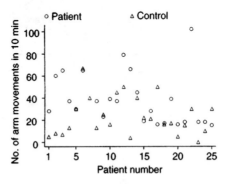

5.4.1   Is this a matched or unmatched case–control study?

5.4.2   The figure plots movement against patient number. Why might this be misleading?

5.4.3   How could the data be plotted more clearly?

ANSWERS

5.3.1 Patient number is not an important variable, it is only an identifier. Using it on the x-axis makes the graph harder to read.

5.3.2 We could do a scatter plot of difference against group (or dot plot), as in the left-hand figure below. Overlapping points are separated by adding some random noise, called 'jittering'. Another possibility would be to plot temperature after typing against temperature before, using separate symbols for the two groups, as in the right-hand figure. The line of equality has been added to each diagram. The points would be scattered about this if the mean change in temperature were zero.

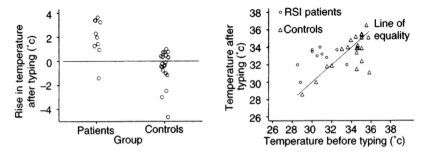

5.4.1 The study is unmatched. Each group is a consecutive series of patients. Thus there is no link between, say, the tenth CHD patient and the tenth control.

5.4.2 Not only does the patient number convey no useful information, but the graph implies that there is matching. The tenth CHD case and the tenth control are in the same vertical line.

5.4.3 A scatter plot of groups would be much better:

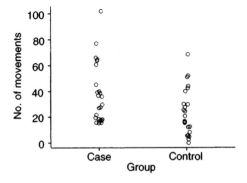

QUESTIONS

5.5 · The relationship between mutant frequency in peripheral lymphocytes and domestic radon concentration was investigated in a small town. Non-smoking subjects were selected from a GP list, non-randomly, so as to give a wide range of radon exposures (Bridges *et al.* 1991). The results are shown in the following figure:

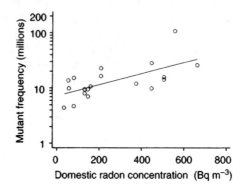

5.5.1   What kind of scale is used on the vertical axis?

5.5.2   What are the effects of such a scale?

5.6   Many prescribed drugs show a seasonal pattern in their use. The following graph shows an example of this and is taken from routinely collected prescribing analyses and cost (PACT) data (Heywood 1991):

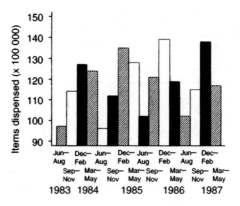

5.6.1   What kind of graph is this?

5.6.2   What feature of the graph might make it misleading?

5.6.3   What feature of the graph makes it difficult to see the pattern?

5.6.4   How could the graph be improved?

ANSWERS

5.5.1   This is a logarithmic scale (*Intro* §5.9).

5.5.2   The effect is to compress the scale for high values and stretch the scale for low values. This may make positively skew distributions symmetrical. If the variability in mutant frequency were greater for samples with high means than for samples with low means, the log scale may make the variation more uniform. It makes multiplicative relationships additive and may straighten curved relationships (*Intro* §5.9).

5.6.1   This is a bar chart (*Intro* §5.5).

5.6.2   The graph has a truncated scale which starts at 90. This will elongate the relevant part of the axis and exaggerate the variation in prescribing (*Intro* §5.8).

5.6.3   The graph presented has used three different shadings for the bars represent the variation across the four seasons. Thus the same season is not always represented by the same shade and so the visual impact of the seasonal pattern is obscured.

5.6.4   An improvement is readily achieved by using four different shadings as shown below. Now the seasonal pattern is clearly displayed. We have replaced the truncated scale with a scale which starts at zero.

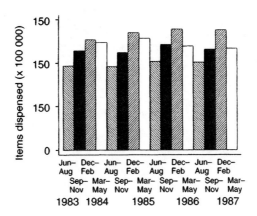

QUESTIONS

5.7   The figure below is based on one given in a paper reporting a study
of depression in patients undergoing cardiac surgery. Patients were
asked to complete several psychometric tests on the day before cardiac surgery, and again on the day before discharge from hospital. The
tests included the Centre for Epidemiological Studies Depression Scale
(CES-D) and the Spielberger Trait Anxiety Inventory (STAI-S). The
figure was described as showing gender differences in depression and
anxiety before and after cardiac surgery (Burker *et al.* 1995).

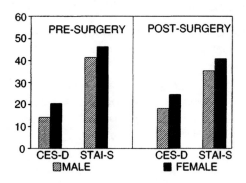

5.7.1   How might the figure be presented to show clearly changes from the
state before surgery to that after surgery?

5.7.2   In what ways might the data be presented if all the data were available,
rather than mean scores?

ANSWERS

5.7.1   The published graph makes a direct comparison between sexes, then between the depression and anxiety scales. What stands out is that men have lower mean scores than women and that STAI-S scores are higher than CES-D. The latter is meaningless, as these scales are not comparable. Comparison of pre- and post-surgery scores is difficult, as the bars are far apart. The figure below shows a different version of the bar chart. The vertical axis has been labelled. The bars have been rearranged so that the most direct comparison is between pre- and post-surgery scores, then between the sexes, showing that depression increases with surgery and anxiety decreases, and that both are higher in women than in men. The pattern of differences between CES-D and STAI-S can be seen clearly. To make it a little easier to read, the upper-case legends have been changed to lower case. The words 'depression' and 'anxiety' have also been added, to remind the reader what these scales are measuring.

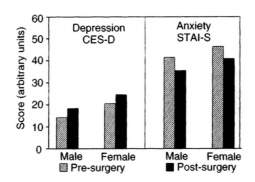

5.7.2   There is no indication of either the variability of the data or the precision of the mean estimates. To indicate the variability, standard deviation lines could be added to the bars in the figure, jutting out of the top of the bars like little television aerials. There are no standard deviations given in the paper, only P values, so we cannot improve the diagram with the information available. If the precision of the estimated means were thought more important, standard error or confidence interval lines could be added instead. We could use a box and whisker plot to do this. We could also use a dot or scatter plot, which would show all the data in each group (*Intro* §5.6). If we wanted to show the means and their standard errors, we could add these to the scatter diagram.

QUESTIONS

5.8   In a case–control study to investigate the relationship between sudden
infant death syndrome and sleeping environment, parental interviews
were conducted for 325 babies who died and 1 300 control infants (Blair
et al. 1999). The usual sleeping environments were compared in a graph
similar to the following:

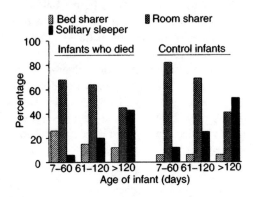

5.8.1   Why is it difficult to compare the sleeping environment of babies who
died and control infants in this graph? How could it be improved?

5.8.2   How could the fact that the percentages of bed sharers, room sharers,
and solitary sleepers add up to 100 be used to simplify the graph?

ANSWERS

5.8.1   The bars which need to be compared, for infants who died and controls
         of the same age, are not close together. It is easier to see the effect of
         age than the difference between cases and controls. Putting the cases
         and controls together makes the comparison easier:

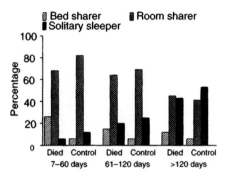

5.8.2   We can put the three sleeping categories one above the other in a stacked
         bar chart. This brings out the consistent excess of bed-sharing among
         the infants who died.

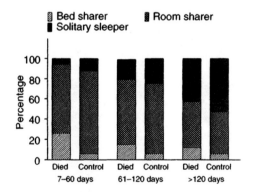

6
Probability

This chapter deals with probability and probability distributions for discrete variables.

Probability is the proportion of occasions on which an event would happen if the circumstances were repeated indefinitely. It lies between 0.0 and 1.0, inclusive. A different way of presenting probability is odds, the probability of the event divided by the probability that the event does not occur.

If we have a set of all possible events which are mutually exclusive (i.e. if one occurs then the others cannot occur) then their probabilities form a probability distribution. The sum of the probabilities is one. These probabilities can be summarized using the mean and variance of the distribution.

The Binomial distribution is a theoretical probability distribution. It arises when the events are successes in a fixed number of independent repetitions of a success or fail trial, such as tossing a coin several times or observing several patients each of whom may survive or die. The number of successes, e.g. heads or survivals, follows a Binomial distribution. This is a family of distributions defined by two parameters, the probability of success, p, and the number of repetitions, n. It has mean np and variance $np(1 - p)$.

The Poisson distribution is the theoretical distribution followed by the number of events in a unit of time, when events happen independently and randomly. Its mean and variance are both equal to the rate at which events happen, the only parameter of the distribution.

A conditional probability is the probability of an event given that some other event has already occurred. It is important not to confuse the probability that event A occurs given event B has occurred with the probability that event B occurs given that event A has occurred, the prosecutor's fallacy.

QUESTIONS

6.1   A Gloucestershire hospital is apparently refusing to tell a couple the sex of their unborn child. A spokesman for the hospital said that it had a policy of not revealing a baby's sex for several reasons, including the possibility of getting it wrong. 'We can only really be accurate in half of cases', he said (Daily Telegraph 1999).

6.1.1   What probability of correctly ascertaining the sex of an unborn child does the spokesman claim?

6.1.2   If a couple simply tossed a coin to guess the sex of their unborn child, saying for example that heads meant male and tails meant female, what is the probability that they would be correct?

6.1.3   Assuming the spokesman is giving correct information, what do you think of the hospital's technique for ascertaining the sex of a fetus?

6.2   A woman wrote to the health page of a magazine asking about the risk of miscarriage. She had lost her first pregnancy, and was worried that the same thing would happen again. The medical correspondent replied that about one in eight pregnancies miscarry, but not because there is anything wrong with the mother or fetus. There is only a 1 in 64 chance of it happening a second time. There was every chance that her next pregnancy would be successful (Smith 1980).

6.2.1   What principle was used in calculating the 1 in 64 chance? What assumption has been made about miscarriages?

6.2.2   Of what is 1 in 64 the probability?

6.2.3   What is the probability that the woman's next pregnancy will miscarry?

6.3   The following appeared in a newspaper article (Bosely 1999) about assisted conception, quoting a consultant in the field:

At his clinic, he says, on the first cycle of fertility treatment, 30% get pregnant 30% do not and drop out, 30% try again. Of those who go for a second treatment, there is a similar split of a successful third, a drop out third, and a try again third. His calculation is that those who persist have an increased chance each time, on the basis that the pool is smaller and yet a third must get pregnant.

Is the calculation correct?

ANSWERS

6.1.1   If they were accurate in half of cases then the probability is a half or 0.5.

6.1.2   If the couple simply tossed a coin they would also be right half of the time i.e. with probability 0.5.

6.1.3   According to the spokesman, the hospital's technique is no better than chance. It seems very likely that the spokesman was misinformed!

6.2.1   This is the multiplication rule of probability, that the probability that two events both happen is the product of their probabilities. The assumption is that miscarriages are independent events, and women who have had one have the same probability of miscarrying the next pregnancy as do women who have not miscarried (*Intro* §6.1).

6.2.2   This is the probability that a woman will have two successive pregnancies miscarry, given the assumption in (6.2.1), and is calculated before the pregnancies have happened (*Intro* §6.2).

6.2.3   One in eight. The first pregnancy has already happened and does not have any probability. One in 64 is the probability that her second and third pregnancies will miscarry. These calculations assume that miscarriages are independent, which may not be true.

6.3   No. If a third must get pregnant, the chance of being in that group is one-third, no matter how many or how few women are 'in the pool' (*Intro* §6.2, 6.8). (This would ignore the possibility that women who fail to conceive the first time may be less likely to conceive at the second attempt than the women who are on the first cycle, and so for them the probability of conception may be less than one-third.)

QUESTIONS

6.4   '20 million-to-1 family' was the headline in *The Mirror*, a British popular newspaper (January 28 1999, p. 3). The story was that a family of eight children had been born in the order girl, boy, girl, boy, girl, boy, girl, boy, and that the odds against this were 20 000 000 to 1. 'To have had a total of four boys and four girls in no specific order would have been amazing enough. But to have had them born in such an order is even more so. The chances of this happening are infinitesimal,' said the proud father.

6.4.1   Is this any more surprising than any other combination and ordering of sexes of children in a family of eight?

6.4.2   How would you calculate both the probability of and odds against this particular order? (For simplicity, we can assume boys and girls are equally likely and births are independent.) Just for a change, try the calculation. What would be the probability of having alternation of sex in eight births? Which properties of probability are you using?

6.4.3   Given the assumptions, what distribution would be followed by the number of girls in eight children? How amazing would four girls and four boys be?

ANSWERS

6.4.1   Each child can be boy or girl. Thus there are

$$2 \times 2 \times 2 \times 2 \times 2 \times 2 \times 2 \times 2 = 256$$

possible arrangements. If births were independent and boys and girls were equally likely, these 256 possible family structures would all be equally likely. Boy, boy, boy, boy, girl, girl, girl, girl would be as likely as the structure observed, and so would be boy, boy, girl, boy, girl, girl, girl, girl.

6.4.2   The probability of any given family structure of eight children would be the same, $1/256 = 0.0039$, and odds against are 255 to 1. The probability that the first birth is a girl is 0.5, as is the probability that the next is a boy. Hence, the probability of a girl followed by a boy is 0.5×0.5, and the probability of four such pairs is

$$0.5 \times 0.5 \times 0.5 \times 0.5 \times 0.5 \times 0.5 \times 0.5 \times 0.5 = 0.0039$$

We used the multiplication rule for independent events. For alternating sexes, we must include the possibility of boy, girl, boy, girl, boy, girl, boy, girl. This and girl, boy, girl, boy, girl, boy, girl, boy are mutually exclusive, so we can add their probabilities to get the probability of alternating sexes as

$$0.0039 + 0.0039 = 0.0078$$

In fact, boys are more likely than girls (approximate ratio $51:49$) and there is a very, very small tendency for parents to have children of the same sex. These would alter the probabilities only very slightly (*Intro* §6.2).

6.4.3   The number of girls would follow Binomial distribution with parameters $n = 8$ and $p = 0.5$. The probability of four girls is given by the Binomial probability formula:

$$\frac{n!}{(n-r)!r!}p^r(1-p)^{n-r} = \frac{8!}{4!4!} \times 0.5^4 \times (1-0.5)^4 = 0.27$$

Thus the occurrence of four girls and four boys is hardly amazing. It would occur in more than a quarter of sibships of eight children (*Intro* §6.4).

QUESTIONS

6.5   A computing magazine reported that one-third of graduates working in
            computing have degrees in information technology (IT) and two-thirds
            have degrees in other subjects. They conclude that 'arts and science
            graduates are twice as likely as IT graduates to pursue careers as IT
            professionals' (*RSS News* June 1999, p. 15).

6.5.1   Why is the conclusion false?

❗ 6.5.2   What medical statistical term would be used to describe the estimate
            'twice as likely'?

❗ 6.5.3   What extra information would be needed to compare the probabilities
            of working in IT for non-IT and IT graduates?

ANSWERS

6.5.1 The probability of being an arts or science graduate given that the graduate works in IT is two-thirds. This is not the same as the probability that a graduate works in IT given a degree in arts or science. This is an example of the prosecutor's fallacy (*Intro3* §6.8).

6.5.2 It is the relative risk of working in IT for non-IT graduates compared to IT graduates.

6.5.3 We would need to know what proportion of graduates have degrees in IT. We could use this to estimate the relative risk of working in IT for IT graduates compared to non-IT graduates. The probabilities are linked by

$$\text{PROB(works in IT if non-IT grad) PROB(non-IT grad)}$$
$$= \text{PROB(non-IT grad if works in IT) PROB(works in IT)}$$

So

$$\text{PROB(works in IT if non-IT grad)}$$
$$= \frac{\text{PROB(non-IT grad if works in IT) PROB(works in IT)}}{\text{PROB(non-IT grad)}}$$

Similarly

$$\text{PROB(works in IT if IT grad)}$$
$$= \frac{\text{PROB(IT grad if works in IT) PROB(works in IT)}}{\text{PROB(IT grad)}}$$

Thus

$$\frac{\text{PROB(works in IT if non-IT grad)}}{\text{PROB(works in IT if IT grad)}}$$
$$= \frac{\text{PROB(non-IT grad if works in IT) PROB(IT grad)}}{\text{PROB(IT grad if works in IT) PROB(non-IT grad)}}$$
$$= \frac{2/3 \ \text{PROB(IT grad)}}{1/3 \ \text{PROB(non-IT grad)}} = 2 \times \frac{\text{PROB(IT grad)}}{\text{PROB(non-IT grad)}}$$

As only a small proportion of graduates are IT graduates, the odds on a graduate being in IT, PROB(IT grad)/PROB(non-IT grad), will be a small number and the probability that a non-IT graduate will enter computing will be only a small fraction of the probability that an IT graduate will do so (*Intro* §6.2, 6.8).

QUESTIONS

6.6   Patients are increasingly exposed to numerical information about the risks of disease and the benefits of treatment. This approach assumes that the numerical information can be correctly interpreted by the patient. To investigate this, a cross-sectional study asked a series of questions relating to general numeracy and specifically to the risk reductions associated with breast cancer screening (mammography) (Schwartz *et al.* 1997).

6.6.1   When asked how many heads they would expect from 1 000 flips of a fair coin, about one-third of women gave answers less than 300, with the most common answers being 25, 50, and 250. What is the correct answer?

A statement was given and the respondents were asked to interpret the information given. What are the correct answers? 'Women who are screened for breast cancer by mammogram have a 33% reduction in the risk of death from the disease in the next 10 years, from a baseline risk of 12 in 1 000'
'Imagine 1 000 women just like you.'

6.6.2   'Of these women, what is your best guess about how many will die from breast cancer during the next 10 years if they are not screened every year for breast cancer by mammogram?'

6.6.3   'Of these women, what is your best guess about how many will die from breast cancer during the next 10 years if they are screened every year for breast cancer by mammogram?'

6.7   In the film The Bridge on the River Kwai (Lean 1957), Jack Hawkins describes to William Holden the risk of parachuting in the following terms: 'If you make one jump you've only got a 50% chance of injury, two jumps 80%, and three jumps you're bound to catch a packet.'

What do you think of this estimate of the probabilities?

6.8   A newspaper letter on the subject of the Royal Ulster Constabulary contained the following: 'Until considerably more than the present 8% of the nationalist community belong to the police force, this will endure.' (Wood 1999).

Do you think that 8% of the population belong to the police force? What do you think the writer meant? What classic fallacy of probability does this illustrate?

ANSWERS

6.6.1   If the coin was fair then the probability of a head would be 0.5 and so the expected number of heads in 1 000 tosses would be $0.5 \times 1\,000 = 500$ (*Intro* §6.2, 6.6).

6.6.2   The baseline risk of death from breast cancer is given as 12 in 1 000 and so the best estimate is that 12 would die in the next 10 years if there was no screening.

6.6.3   Screening reduces the risk of death by 33% so the screened group will have an estimated $(100 - 33)\% \times 12$ deaths, about 8.

6.7   It seems unlikely that the risk of the jump would actually increase with the number of jumps. If the risk stayed the same at 50%, the probability of an injury in two jumps would be the sum of the probability of being injured in the first jump (0.5) plus the probability of not being injured in the first jump (0.5) times the probability of being injured in the second (0.5), giving $0.5 + 0.5 \times 0.5 = 0.75$. For three jumps the probability of injury would be $0.5 + 0.5 \times 0.5 + 0.5 \times 0.5 \times 0.5 = 0.875$, pretty high but not as bad as 'bound to', which presumably means probability 1.0 (*Intro* §6.2, *Intro3* §6.8). If parachuting were really that dangerous, we doubt that anyone would do it, even in wartime.

6.8   It cannot be that 8% of the population belong to the police. This would be about one-third of men of working age! He meant that 8% of the police force belong to the nationalist community. This is an example of the prosecutor's fallacy, confusing the probability of A (nationalist community) given B (police force) with the probability of B (police force) given A (nationalist community) (*Intro* §6.2, *Intro3* §6.8).

7
The Normal distribution

When we have a continuous variable we represent the probability distribution using probability density, rather than probability. Probability is attached not to particular values of the variable but to sets of values, such as all the possible values between two numbers. It can be represented as the area under part of a probability density curve.

The Normal distribution is the most important probability distribution in statistics. It is a continuous distribution to which the Binomial distribution converges as the number of trials increases and the Poisson distribution converges as its mean increases. The Normal is a family of distributions defined by two parameters, its mean μ ('mu') and variance σ^2 ('sigma squared'). The Standard Normal distribution has mean zero and variance one. Its probabilities are given in tables. If we have any set of independent identically distributed variables, their mean and sum tend to Normal distributions as the number of variables increases (the central limit theorem). Many things which we calculate from samples, such as means and proportions, tend to follow a Normal distribution as the sample size increases. Many naturally occurring variables, or their logarithms, follow a Normal distribution.

Many statistical methods require that data follow a Normal distribution at least approximately. Graphical methods such as histograms and Normal plots can be used to check this assumption.

QUESTIONS

7.1   Fatigue scores were obtained from 15 283 subjects drawn from GP lists. These were found by scoring the answers to a series of questions as 0, 1, 2, or 3 and adding to give a total score. A graph similar to this was presented:

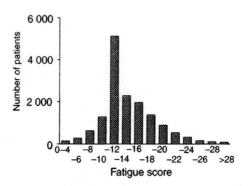

The authors said that since there was a large number of subjects the distributions of responses to the fatigue and the GHQ (see Question 4.3) follow a Normal distribution (Pawlikowska *et al.* 1994).

7.1.1   What is the shape of this frequency distribution?

7.1.2   Does the fatigue score follow a Normal distribution?

7.1.3   Does the sample size influence whether the data follow a Normal distribution?

7.2   The table below shows data from a study of semen analysis and donor success in a programme of artificial insemination by donor (AID) (Paraskevaides *et al.* 1991). From the data presented, do you think it likely that semen count and % motility have Normal distributions?

Semen indices in most and least fertile donors

	Successful donors		Unsuccessful donors	
	No.	Mean (SD)	No.	Mean (SD)
Semen count (10^6/ml)	18	146.4 (95.7)	19	124.8 (81.8)
% motility	17	60.7 (9.7)	19	58.5 (12.8)

7.3   In a consumer column in a daily newspaper, a reader asked why the waist measurement in men's ready-to-wear trousers tended to be an even number while the inside leg measurement tended to be an odd number. Another reader replied that a shop assistant had told him that 'most men had legs an odd number of inches long' (*The Guardian* 1998). Why could the shop assistant not be right?

ANSWERS

7.1.1 There is a long tail on the right, so the distribution is skew to the right or positively skew.

7.1.2 No, the distribution of fatigue score is skew, whereas the Normal distribution is symmetrical. Also, the fatigue scores can take only integer values, whereas the Normal distribution is continuous. As there are quite a lot of possible values, the latter would not matter for most purposes.

7.1.3 The size of the sample does not affect the shape of distribution. It may affect our ability to tell whether data are consistent with a Normal distribution, which these appear not to be. It also affects whether the assumption that the data follow a Normal distribution, which some statistical methods require, is important.

7.2 For data that follow a Normal distribution, 2.5% of the observations will lie below the mean minus 2 standard deviations. Here this would imply negative values for semen count, which are impossible. Hence we conclude that it is unlikely that semen count follows a Normal distribution. With % motility, the standard deviation is much less than half the mean and so the mean minus 2 standard deviations is a possible value. Hence the data could follow a Normal distribution but without seeing all of the observations we cannot be sure. Below we show Normal distributions for both semen count and % motility with the same means and standard deviations as the data (*Intro* §7.4).

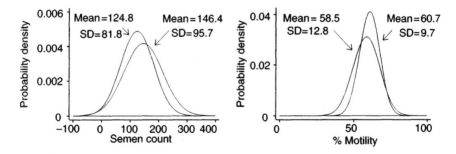

7.3 Inside leg length is a continuous measurement which follows an approximately Normal distribution. Hence inside leg length could take any value between a certain range. The value of the measurement depends on the accuracy to which it is measured. With a tape measure it is common to measure to the nearest inch giving a value which could be even or odd. If the measurement was to the nearest two inches then of course only even or odd values would be found. However, it is not common practice to do this (*Intro* §7.4).

QUESTIONS

7.4   The report of a clinical trial in ophthalmology contained the following
statement about the statistical methods used: 'For continuous variables,
the mean was compared using a non-paired t test after checking for
normality using an inverse normal plot.' (Damji *et al.* 1999).

✚ 7.4.1   What is an 'inverse normal plot'?

The authors did not show their plots in the paper, but as they included
all their data, and as they used Stata for their analysis, we can recon-
struct them. Here are the intraocular pressures measured at baseline:

17	20	21	23	24	26
18	20	22	23	25	26
18	20	22	23	25	27
18	20	22	23	25	28
19	20	22	23	26	29
19	20	22	23	26	30

Here is the plot for these data:

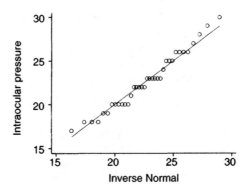

✚ 7.4.2   Do you think that the data were from a Normal distribution? If not,
how do they differ?

ANSWERS

7.4.1   An inverse normal plot, usually shortened to 'normal plot', is used to
        see whether data could come from a Normal distribution. We order
        the data, then plot the observations against the values which we would
        expect from a sample of the same size from a Normal distribution. If
        the data are from a Normal distribution, the observations will lie on a
        straight line (*Intro* §7.5).

7.4.2   The points lie very close to the straight line. Because the data are given
        to the nearest integer and there are only a few possible values the data
        are grouped, causing the short horizontal series of points in the plot.
        The points curve very slightly upwards away from the line at the top
        and bottom, suggesting a very small amount of skewness (*Intro* §7.5).
        Neither of these would upset the t test (*Intro* §10.5).

QUESTIONS

7.5   Sperm concentration is found by counting the number of sperm in a small, fixed volume of semen, then multiplying by a constant to give an estimated count of sperm per litre of semen. Bromwich *et al.* (1994) studied the shape of the distribution of sperm concentration. They considered the Uniform, Normal, and Lognormal as possible shapes.

7.5.1   Which of these possible distributions do you think least likely for a biological measurement?

They gave the following histogram of sperm concentration in semen samples provided by men presenting for *in vitro* fertilization:

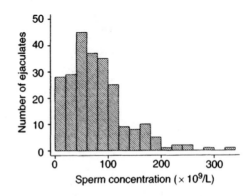

7.5.2   What shape does this distribution have?

➕ 7.5.3   The authors suggest that this distribution may be Lognormal. How could graphical methods be used to investigate this?

➕ 7.5.4   What type of distribution might counts be expected to follow?

❗➕ 7.5.5   How might we investigate the fit to this distribution here, remembering that the counts have been multiplied by an unknown constant?

ANSWERS

7.5.1   The Uniform is least likely because it has no tails. Distributions of bio-
         logical measurements usually have tails. Many variables follow Normal
         and Lognormal distributions.

7.5.2   The distribution is skew to the right (longer tail on the right) or posi-
         tively skew.

7.5.3   They could take the logs of the observations and plot a Normal distribu-
         tion curve on the histogram. They could also construct a Normal plot
         of the log sperm concentrations. We have approximated their data from
         the histogram and done this for the log-transformed data. Clearly the
         log-transformed data are negatively skew and we do not have a Lognor-
         mal distribution:

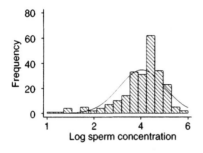 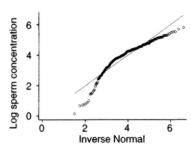

7.5.4   Counts often follow a Poisson distribution.

7.5.5   We cannot use the exact probabilities or mean and variance of the Pois-
         son distribution, because the original counts have been multiplied by
         an unknown constant. We can use the fact that a square root trans-
         formation is the transformation which will make a Poisson distribution
         Normal. If the square root is Normal, the observations may have a dis-
         tribution related to the Poisson. Below are a histogram and Normal plot
         for the square root of the sperm concentrations. The fit to the Normal is
         much better than for either the untransformed or log-transformed data.
         We can conclude that there is good evidence that a Poisson distribution
         may underlie the distribution of sperm concentration.

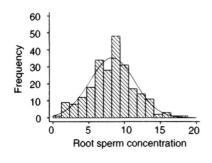 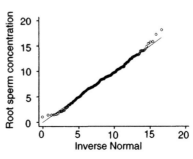

8
Estimation

This chapter covers standard errors and confidence intervals, and their application to some large sample problems.

Standard errors are used in statistical inference, which means using a sample to answer a question about the population from which it is drawn. Samples are used to produce estimates for populations. These vary from sample to sample. The estimates from all possible samples of a given size form the sampling distribution of the estimate. Standard error is the standard deviation of the sampling distribution. It measures how good the estimate is. It is usually estimated from the data. It is roughly proportional to one over the square root of the sample size. The standard error of a mean is $s/\sqrt{n}$ and of a proportion $\sqrt{p(1-p)/n}$.

We often denote the mean of a population by μ and the standard deviation by σ. We use a sample to estimate quantities such as these in the whole population. We can use a single number, such as the mean, calculated from the sample as an estimate. This is called a point estimate. It will not be exactly the same as the population value (e.g. mean). It is useful in addition to find an interval estimate, a range of values which we hope will include the population value. This is usually a 95% confidence interval. A 95% confidence interval is a range of values chosen so that the population value would lie within the confidence intervals calculated from 95% of possible samples. It therefore reflects the amount by which population estimates vary from sample to sample. Other probabilities can be used, e.g. 90% or 99%. A bigger probability leads to a wider interval, a smaller probability to a narrower interval with more risk of being wrong. Standard errors are often used to calculate confidence intervals.

Standard error and confidence interval are often abbreviated to SE and CI. Standard errors and confidence intervals can be calculated for anything obtained from a sample. It is easy to do this for the differences between two means and between two proportions. Provided the sample is large enough, the confidence interval is found from the estimate ±1.96 standard errors.

For some small sample problems, the confidence interval is better based on the individual probabilities of the distribution, rather than a large sample approximation. Binomial proportions and Poisson rates are examples.

QUESTIONS

8.1   A UK study of factors affecting the outcome of pregnancy among 1 513
women reported that the overall incidence of pre-term births was 7.5%,
SE = 0.68%, 95% CI 6.1 to 8.8% (Peacock *et al.* 1995).

8.1.1   What is meant by SE = 0.68%?

8.1.2   What is meant by 95% CI 6.1 to 8.8%?

8.1.3   What two distributions are used to calculate the SE and the CI?

8.1.4   How would the confidence interval change if 90% limits were used?

8.1.5   How would the confidence interval change if 99% limits were used?

8.1.6   Another study conducted at about the same time in Denmark and
including 51 851 women, reported that the overall incidence of pre-term
birth was 4.5% (95% CI 4.3 to 4.7%). Explain why this 95% CI is narrower than that reported in the UK study. Do you think that there is
a real difference in pre-term birth rates between the two populations
being studied?

ANSWERS

8.1.1   This is the standard error. Estimates of population values vary from sample to sample and therefore have a theoretical distribution, the sampling distribution. The standard error of an estimate is a measure of the variability of this distribution. The standard error is the standard deviation of the sampling distribution of the sample estimate. The standard error therefore provides information about the precision of the estimate and is used to calculate confidence intervals around the estimates. Here the value of 0.68 is the standard error of the percentage of pre-term births. The units of the standard error is the same as for the sample estimate and hence is in percentage points (*Intro* §8.2, 8.4).

8.1.2   This is the 95% CI. It is a range of values which we estimate will contain the population percentage of pre-term births. This is in the sense that if a large number of samples were taken from the same population, then 95% of the calculated confidence intervals would contain the population percentage. Here, we can deduce that the population value is very likely to lie between 6.1% and 8.8% (*Intro* §8.3).

8.1.3   The sample proportion of pre-term births follows the Binomial distribution and this is therefore used to calculate the standard error. There are 113 pre-term births out of 1 513 and so the distribution of the sample proportion, the Binomial, can be approximated by the Normal. This distribution is used here to calculate the confidence interval (*Intro* §8.4).

8.1.4   If 90% limits were used the confidence interval would be narrower and fewer (90% rather than 95%) of confidence intervals from possible samples would contain the population incidence. Thus the estimated range of possible values would be narrower but there would be more chance of being wrong. (The 90% confidence limits would be 6.4 to 8.6%) (*Intro* §8.3).

8.1.5   If 99% limits were used the confidence interval would be wider and more (99%) of confidence intervals from possible samples would contain the population incidence. Thus there would be less chance of being wrong but the range of possible population values would be greater (the 99% confidence limits would be 5.8 to 9.2%) (*Intro* §8.3).

8.1.6   The Danish study included many more subjects than the UK study and so the estimate of pre-term birth incidence is much more precise. Hence, the 95% CI is narrower. The percentage pre-term in the UK study is 3 percentage points higher than in the Danish study and the two 95% CIs do not overlap. Hence there is some evidence for a real difference (*Intro* §8.3).

QUESTIONS

8.2   One hundred and forty-one babies who developed cerebral palsy were
             compared to a control group of babies made up from the two babies
             immediately after each cerebral palsy baby in the hospital delivery book.
             Hospital notes were reviewed by a researcher who was blind to the baby's
             outcome. Failure to respond to signs of fetal distress was noted in 25.8%
             of the cerebral palsy babies and in 7.1% of the delivery book babies.
             The difference was 18.7 percentage points, with standard error 4.2 and
             95% CI 10.5 to 26.9 percentage points (Gaffney *et al.* 1994).

8.2.1   What is meant by 'the difference was 18.7 percentage points'?

8.2.2   What can we conclude from the 95% CI?

8.3   In a study of bone density and falls in older women, 118 volunteers were
             randomized to receive either calcium supplements plus a program of
             exercise classes or to calcium alone for 2 years. Twelve subjects dropped
             out from the calcium group and 14 from the calcium group taking exer-
             cise, leaving 92 subjects who completed the two year project. The per-
             centage change in bone mineral content and bone mineral density in
             two years was calculated for each individual. The authors reported that
             for the ultradistal forearm the change in bone mineral content was −2.6
             (95% CI −4.6 to −0.6) in the calcium only group and 1.14 (95% CI −0.8
             to 3.1) in the calcium group taking exercise (McMurdo *et al.* 1997).

8.3.1   What do the confidence intervals for the change in bone mineral content
             mean? To what population do they refer?

8.3.2   Confidence intervals are presented for each group separately. Suggest a
             more informative confidence interval. To which population would this
             relate?

8.3.3   Twenty-six out of 114 subjects dropped out. Is there anything the
             authors should have done about them apart from encouraging them
             to continue with the treatment?

ANSWERS

8.2.1   Failure to respond to signs of fetal distress was noted in 25.8% of the cerebral palsy babies and in 7.1% of the delivery book babies. The difference between these two percentages is $25.8 - 7.1 = 18.7$. This is the actual difference in the two percentages and so is expressed in percentage points. This distinguishes it from a relative difference where we might, for example, say that the rate in the delivery book babies was 28% (7.1/25.8) of the rate among the cerebral palsy babies (*Intro* §8.6).

8.2.2   The 95% CI shows that the difference between the two groups is estimated to be at least as large as 10.5 percentage points and may be as great as 26.9 percentage points. Since the interval excludes 0.0, there is good evidence for a real difference in the population from which the samples come (*Intro* §8.6).

8.3.1   The two confidence intervals give us a range of values within which the mean change is estimated to lie in the whole population of women who would volunteer if they were to receive the treatment for that group. The confidence interval for the calcium only group tells us that the mean percentage change is a reduction in bone mineral content somewhere between 0.6 and 4.6 percentage points. For the calcium plus exercise group taking the mean percentage change could be a reduction of 0.8 percentage points or an increase of 3.1 percentage points or any value between these limits. These women were volunteers and it is therefore difficult to extrapolate the findings to a general population (*Intro* §8.3).

8.3.2   The confidence intervals provide estimates of the mean change in bone density over 2 years. Since we are here interested in any effect of exercise on this, a confidence interval for the difference between the two groups would be more useful than the two separate intervals provided. Using the data given the difference in mean change is 3.7 with an approximate 95% CI 0.9 to 6.5. This would still relate to the population of volunteers but since the women were randomized to two groups, we might reasonably expect the sample difference to be representative of all women (*Intro* §8.6, 8.10).

8.3.3   Drop-outs are inevitable in randomized trials. We need to know if there were more drop-outs in one group than the other. It would be helpful to know when the subjects dropped out and to know if it were possible to take any measurements from them. If these measurements were available then an intention to treat analysis could have been performed. If those who dropped out were lost to follow up, some indication of their baseline characteristics would help to assess the effect of leaving them out of the analysis (*Intro* §2.5).

QUESTIONS

8.4   In a study of factors affecting birthweight, blood cotinine level was used to estimate passive smoke exposure among non-smokers. The study reported that the difference in mean birthweight between non-smokers below the lowest and above the highest quintiles of cotinine was 7 g (95% CI −84 to 98 g). Pooling the results of 10 previous studies plus this one gave an estimated difference in mean birthweight between women unexposed and exposed to passive smoke of 31 g (95% CI 19 to 44) (note: mean birthweight is usually about 3 500 g) (Peacock *et al.* 1998).

8.4.1   What does the data from the study show about the effects of passive smoke exposure on birthweight?

8.4.2   How is this information changed when the data are pooled with that from other studies?

8.5   In a randomized trial of alteplase vs streptokinase in acute myocardial infarction, the relative risk of death or severe left ventricular damage was 1.04, 95% CI 0.95 to 1.13 (Anonymous 1990).

8.5.1   What is meant by relative risk? How would it be calculated here?

8.5.2   How was the 95% CI calculated?

8.6   In a prospective study of serum sialic acid concentration and cardiovascular mortality, 54 385 men and women aged 40–74 were followed over 20 years. There were 4 420 deaths due to cardiovascular disease and 4 526 non-cardiovascular deaths. The quartiles of sialic acid concentration were used to divide the men into four equal groups. The relative risk associated with the highest fourth of sialic acid concentration compared to the lowest fourth was 2.38 (95% CI 2.01 to 2.83) (Lindberg *et al.* 1991).

8.6.1   What is meant by relative risk 2.38?

8.6.2   What method could be used to calculate it in this study?

ANSWERS

8.4.1 The study shows that the mean birthweight of babies for women exposed to low levels of passive smoke during pregnancy is estimated to be 7 g more than the mean birthweight for women heavily exposed to passive smoke. The 95% CI shows that in the population, mean birthweight for women with light passive smoke exposure might be up to 98 g more than those heavily exposed or mean birthweight could be 84 g less (*Intro* §8.5).

8.4.2 The single study suggests that the effect of passive smoking on birthweight is very small. The 95% CI is wide reflecting imprecision in the estimation of the passive smoke effect. The pooled result gives a mean difference which is slightly bigger. The 95% CI for the difference shows that the population difference is now more precisely estimated as lying between 19 and 44 g. This shows the gain in precision obtained by pooling data from several studies and suggests that there is a real but small adverse effect (*Intro* §8.3). (See question 17.10 for further discussion of this study.)

8.5.1 The risk is the probability that an individual will die or have severe damage. Relative risk is the ratio of the risk in the alteplase group to that in the streptokinase group. If the risk is equal in the two groups then the relative risk will be one. A value over one indicates an increased risk in the first group compared to the second and a value below one indicates a reduced risk in the first group. Here the relative risk is simply the ratio of the proportions dying or damaged in the two groups (*Intro* §8.6).

8.5.2 This is calculated from the sample so that for 95% of samples the confidence interval will include the population value. Here it can be calculated from the standard error of the log relative risk, using a large sample Normal approximation (*Intro* §8.6).

8.6.1 Risk is the probability that an individual will experience the event, here death. Relative risk is the ratio of the risk among those with the factor (high sialic acid) to the risk of death among those without the factor (low sialic acid). The relative risk tells us that the risk of death is 2.38 times as great in those with high sialic acid compared to those with low sialic acid (*Intro* §8.6).

8.6.2 This is a cohort study where we start with the risk factor (sialic acid) and so we can calculate the risks directly and hence obtain the ratio of risks (*Intro* §8.6).

9
Significance tests

Significance tests are a way of using the sample to tell us something about the population from which it came, a process called statistical inference. They are used to test a proposition, such as 'two populations have the same mean'.

A P value is the result of a significance test. It measures the strength of the evidence concerning some proposition about the populations. The null hypothesis is stated, that there is no relationship or difference in the population from which the sample is drawn. A test statistic is found which would follow a known distribution if the null hypothesis were true. P is the probability of a test statistic as far from what would be expected as that observed, if the null hypothesis were true. If P is small, usually taken to be less than 0.05, we have evidence against the null hypothesis. The smaller P is, the stronger is the evidence. If the probability of a value as extreme as that observed is high we have weak evidence against the null hypothesis, the data are consistent with the null hypothesis and the relationship or difference is not significant. If the difference is not significant we have failed to show that there is a difference in the population, but one may still exist. The sample may not be large enough to detect it. We have *not* proved that there is no difference.

Because there is a chance of getting a significant result when the null hypothesis is true, doing many related tests increases our chance of producing a spurious result. We can correct for this in several ways, such as the Bonferroni correction or by specially planned sequential tests.

If the 95% CI for a statistic such as a difference between two means excludes the value the statistic would have under the null hypothesis, the difference is significant at the 5% level. Null hypothesis values are usually zero for a difference, one for a ratio, etc. Sometimes the null hypothesis changes the calculation of standard errors, those derived from the Binomial and Poisson distributions for example. In these cases there may be a better significance test than that based on the confidence interval not including the null value. When this happens the confidence interval and significance test may not be entirely consistent.

QUESTIONS

9.1   In a double-blind comparison of two ointments, containing calcipotriol
           or betamethasone, for the treatment of psoriasis, 345 subjects were given
           one ointment on the left side of the body and the other on the right, the
           side being chosen at random. The severity of the condition was assessed
           in terms of a score. The score was significantly lower ($P < 0.001$) for
           the calcipotriol side than the betamethasone side.

9.1.1   What is meant by '$P < 0.001$'?

           The sample size was calculated to allow detection of a difference of
           5% between treatments in mean change in score, assuming a standard
           deviation for change in score of 25%, a type I error of 0.05 (alpha = 5%,
           two-tailed) and a type II error of 0.10 (power = 90%) (Kragballe *et al.*
           1991).

9.1.2   What is meant by type I error and type II error?

9.2   In a randomized trial of morphine versus placebo for the anaesthesia of
           mechanically ventilated pre-term babies, it was reported that morphine-
           treated babies showed a significant reduction in adrenaline concentra-
           tions during the first 24 hours (median change -0.4 nmol/L, $P < 0.001$),
           which was not seen in the placebo group (median change 0.2 nmol/L,
           $P = 0.79$) (Quinn *et al.* 1993).

9.2.1   What is wrong with this approach to the analysis?

9.2.2   Suggest a better method.

ANSWERS

9.1.1   This is the result of a significance test. P is the probability of getting a difference as far from expectation as that observed when the null hypothesis is in fact true. Here the null hypothesis is that there is no difference between the two treatments as measured by a visual assessment. P is very small showing that the probability of the observed difference occurring if there is really no difference between the treatments was small. We say that the difference is statistically significant and conclude that there is good evidence for a difference between the treatments in the whole population (*Intro* §9.3).

9.1.2   A type I error is when we get a significant result when the null hypothesis is true. The probability of a type I error is equal to the P value. The maximum type I error probability is set in advance, usually 0.05 (*Intro* §9.4).

A type II error occurs when we get a non-significant result when the null hypothesis is false. In other words, we fail to detect a real difference. The probability of a type II error depends on the size of the difference in the population, as well as on the sample size and the significance level chosen (*Intro* §9.4).

9.2.1   The authors are looking at each group separately, testing the null hypothesis that there is no change in adrenaline. If we compare in this way, we are wrongly interpreting a non-significant result as meaning that there is no effect.

9.2.2   It would be much better to compare the two groups directly, testing the null hypothesis that the change is the same in the two groups. This could be done by the large sample Normal comparison of two means (*Intro* §9.7).

QUESTIONS

9.3   In a double-blind, randomized-controlled trial, children with mild croup were allocated to receive a single dose of an oral steroid (dexamethasone) or placebo (Geelhoed *et al.* 1996). The results were reported as follows:

Outcome measures for children with mild croup treated with steroid or placebo. Except where stated otherwise, values are means (standard deviation)

	Steroid	Placebo	Significance
Number followed up	48	48	
Number who reattended with croup	0	8	P < 0.01
Number admitted with croup	0	1	NS
Number who reattended for other reasons	18	18	NS
Duration of croup symptoms (days)	1.7 (1.8)	2 (1.6)	NS
Duration of viral symptoms (days)	6.5 (4.4)	6.7 (4.2)	NS

NS = Not significant.

9.3.1   How could 'NS' be more usefully reported?

9.3.2   What additional information would a confidence interval provide for the comparison of duration between the two groups?

9.4   Twenty-five breast cancer patients were given 50 Gy in fractions of 2 Gy over 5 weeks. Lung function was measured initially, at 1 week, at 3 months and at 1 year (Lund *et al.* 1991). The aim of the study was to see whether lung function was lowered following radiotherapy. Some results are shown in the table.

Paired t test analyses of difference in forced vital capacity (FVC) (ml) between first and subsequent visits

	Difference in FVC between visits		
	$2-1$ ($n = 25$)	$3-1$ ($n = 24$)	$4-1$ ($n = 23$)
Mean	48	−63	−49
SD	210	158	266
SEM	42	32	55
P(1-sided)	0.13	0.032	0.19

9.4.1   What is meant by 'P (1-sided)'?

❶ 9.4.2   Why is P = 0.13 wrong, assuming there is no misprint in the table?

❶ 9.4.3   Is a one-sided test justified here, and what would be the effect of using a two-sided test?

❶ 9.4.4   The authors reported that 'a small but statistically significant reduction appeared after 3 months but disappeared within one year.' Comment on this statement.

ANSWERS

9.3.1   The actual P value would be more helpful even if it is bigger than 0.05 and hence non-significant, since the P value shows the weight of evidence against the null hypothesis. A P value close to 0.05 would provide more evidence against the null hypothesis than a P value well above 0.05. This could only be judged if the actual value was given.

9.3.2   A confidence interval for the difference in means would give an estimate of the range of values which the difference between the groups might take in the population. This would be more informative than either a P value alone or a P value and the observed difference. It would enable the reader to judge the precision of the findings and thus be better equipped to interpret them (*Intro* §9.6).

9.4.1   P(1-sided) is the P value from a one-sided test of significance. Because the test is one-sided the null hypothesis must be that the difference is zero or that it is positive. The alternative hypothesis is that the difference is negative, i.e. that FVC goes down between visits. P is thus the probability of getting a reduction in FVC as big as that observed or bigger if, in the population, FVC remained the same or increased (*Intro* §9.5).

9.4.2   P = 0.13 is wrong because the mean difference is positive indicating that FVC increased between visits 1 and 2. Since tests are one-sided, the P value for a positive difference must be bigger than 0.5. If a two-sided test were used the P values would all be doubled and none would be significant.

9.4.3   It is strange to use one-sided tests because these effectively regard a rise in FVC as equivalent to no change and thus non-significant. In practice, one would wish to know if there was a beneficial or harmful effect of radiotherapy. One-sided tests will only detect a harmful effect (*Intro* §9.5).

9.4.4   The size of the reduction is less after one-year (visit 4) than after 3 months (visit 3). The reduction has not disappeared but has become smaller and hence non-significant. Not significant does not mean that there is no difference and so we cannot conclude that FVC at 1 year was the same as at the outset. One would need to follow these patients up for longer to see if their FVC did in fact return to the initial levels (*Intro* §9.6).

QUESTIONS

9.5   In a study of cancer and atmospheric nuclear weapons tests, exposed
            servicemen and civilian nuclear weapons workers were compared to a
            control group matched for age and occupation. One-sided tests and
            90% CIs were used to compare the exposed group to the control group.
            The tests were done in the direction of the observed difference. The
            exposed groups were compared to the general population using stan-
            dardized mortality ratios (SMRs). Two-sided tests and 95% CIs were
            used to compare the exposed group to the general population (Darby
            et al. 1993).

❗ 9.5.1   What problems are there in this approach to testing?

❗ 9.5.2   What two-sided test would be equivalent to a one-sided test at the 5%
            level in the direction of the difference?

9.6   In a study of treatments for menorrhagia during menstruation, 76
            women were randomized to one of three drugs (Bonnar and Sheppard
            1996). The effects of the drugs were measured within the subjects by
            comparing three control menstrual cycles and three treatment menstrual
            cycles in each woman. The women were given no treatment during the
            control cycles. In each subject the control cycles were the three cycles
            preceding the treatment cycles. The authors reported that patients
            treated with ethamsylate used the same number of sanitary towels as in
            the control cycles. A significant reduction in the number of sanitary tow-
            els used was found in patients treated with mefenamic acid (P < 0.05)
            and tranexamic acid (P < 0.01) comparing the control periods with the
            treatment periods. The table below shows some of the results.

Effect of three drugs on duration of bleeding and sanitary towel usage

	Ethamsylate	Mefenamic acid	Tranexamic acid
Mean duration (days) (SD)			
Control	5.7 (1.1)	5.8 (1.3)	5.5 (1.4)
Treatment	5.7 (2.0)	5.3 (1.3)	4.9 (1.8)
Mean no. of sanitary towels (SD)			
Control	25 (9.0)	25 (7.0)	23 (7.0)
Treatment	25 (9.0)	23 (9.0)	20 (6.0)

❗ 9.6.1   What problems are there in the design of this study?

❗ 9.6.2   What problems are there in the analysis?

ANSWERS

9.5.1   In a one-sided test, the alternative hypothesis is that there is a difference in a specified direction. The null hypothesis is then that there is no difference or a difference in the opposite direction. This is reasonable if a difference in the opposite direction would have the same meaning or result in the same action as would no difference.

For the comparison with the control group, this argument does not hold. There is no *a priori* reason to suppose that the exposed group would be any different in cancer risk than the controls. In fact, the controls were chosen so that the risk would be the same, apart from any risk due to the exposure. Thus, an excess of cancer in the control group would be very surprising and lead us to conclude either that radiation exposure protected against cancer or that the groups were not comparable. If we found no difference, on the other hand, we would conclude that there was no evidence that the radiation influenced cancer risk. The conclusions would be different and a one-sided test in the direction of more cancers in the exposed group cannot be justified. It is even harder to justify a one-sided test in the direction of fewer cancers in the exposed group, opposite to the research hypothesis.

For the comparison to the general population, it could be argued that the exposed group, predominantly servicemen, are selected and would have a reduced cancer risk, a phenomenon known as the 'healthy worker effect'. A one-sided test in the direction of more cancers in the exposed group would be arguable, because if radiation had no effect the number of cancers in the exposed group would be the same as or less than that in the general population (*Intro* §9.5).

9.5.2   To test in the direction of the observed difference is in fact to carry out tests in both directions simultaneously. As one of these tests assumes that fewer cancers in the controls is equivalent to no difference, and the other assumes that more cancers in the controls is equivalent to no difference, the tests are contradictory. The procedure is the same as a two-sided test at the 10% level, and is not truly one-sided at all (*Intro* §9.5).

9.6.1   The control cycles were the three cycles preceding the treatment cycles, thus there was no placebo and so the assessment could not be blind. Hence there could be assessment bias. It would have been better to have included placebo cycles in a randomized design (*Intro* §2.6, 2.9).

9.6.2   In this table, the effect of each drug has been analysed for each treatment separately, calculating the difference between the control and the treatment cycles. A comparison between treatments would have been more informative than the within treatment tests presented. This would have indicated if there were any differences between the drugs (*Intro* §9.3).

QUESTIONS

9.7 In a study of bone density and falls in older women, 118 volunteers were randomized to receive either calcium supplements plus a program of exercise classes or to calcium alone for 2 years (McMurdo *et al.* 1997).

9.7.1 The authors reported that they found no significant differences between the groups at baseline. Why were these tests of significance unnecessary?

! 9.7.2 The authors stated that 'the difference between the groups in the number of women falling during the whole 2-year period was not significant (P = 0.158), but between 12 months and 18 months into the study the difference was significant (P = 0.011)'. Does the 'P = 0.011' add anything of value to the results of this study?

9.8 A cohort study investigated the association between back pain and ischaemic heart disease. Eight thousand eight hundred and sixteen Finnish farmers aged 30–66 were followed up for 13 years and cardiac events were noted. The following results were presented:

Age-specific mortality (per 1 000 people and 13 years) of men according to history of back pain

	Back pain	No back pain	P value
Age 30–49 years at start			
Cause of death	($n = 1\,274$)	($n = 586$)	
Ischaemic heart disease	18.1	3.4	0.02
Stroke	0.8	0.0	0.68
Other cardiovascular disease	3.9	5.1	0.49
All causes	56.5	44.4	0.32
Age 50–66 years at start			
Cause of death	($n = 1\,212$)	($n = 576$)	
Ischaemic heart disease	54.5	72.5	0.15
Stroke	7.4	8.1	0.99
Other cardiovascular disease	22.3	26.2	0.74
All causes	169.6	203.6	0.10

In women no association between back pain and any vascular disease was found. The author concluded that back pain may be an early manifestation of atherosclerosis, which leads to ischaemic heart disease (Penttinen 1994).

9.8.1 Which subjects are missing from the table?

9.8.2 How many tests of significance do you think the author did?

9.8.3 How many significant relationships would you expect to find by chance in that number of tests if all the null hypotheses were true?

! 9.8.4 What would you conclude from the significant difference in younger men?

⊕ 9.8.5 How could we use these P values so as to test the null hypothesis that back pain is unrelated to mortality?

ANSWERS

9.7.1   As the subjects were allocated at random to one of two groups, any differences in the characteristics of the groups would have occurred by chance, by definition of randomization. Therefore, the null hypothesis is true and so tests of significance would be meaningless.

9.7.2   This is multiple testing. If we keep testing the data as we collect them, the chance of a spurious significant difference increases. In other words, if the null hypothesis were true, the probability of a significant result would not be 0.05 but something bigger. We therefore test only at the end of the study. The intermediate test does not mean anything (*Intro* §9.10).

9.8.1   The females are missing from the table. These comprised half the sample and we are told that no association was observed among this group.

9.8.2   Eight tests were performed among men and we assume that the same number were done for the women making 16 in all. There may have been other tests as well, using both age groups combined and both sexes combined.

9.8.3   We would expect 5% of tests to be significant by chance if the null hypothesis were true. Hence, with 16 tests we would expect 0.8 tests i.e. about one test to be significant by chance (*Intro* §9.10).

9.8.4   From the table there is no evidence for an association between back pain and stroke or other cardiovascular disease among the younger men. In older men, those with back pain have lower risks than those without back pain for all causes of death. In addition, no associations were observed among women. Thus, it seems likely that the observed association among younger men is a spurious significant result which has arisen because of multiple testing (*Intro* §9.10). If you calculate the actual numbers of death from the rates given in the table, and from these assemble a table for all men, you will find that there is a very slight excess of deaths in each category for men without a history of back pain!

9.8.5   We could use the Bonferroni method. This would require us to calculate the number of relevant tests done, here at least 16. We would then multiply the P values by this. If any P value is below 0.05, the relationship is significant. If our initial hypothesis were specifically about ischaemic heart disease, we would have four tests only, and the relationship between IHD and back pain in younger men would have $P = 4 \times 0.02 = 0.08$, not significant (*Intro* §9.10).

10
Comparing the means of small samples

The t distribution is used to find confidence interval and to do tests of significance for data which follow a Normal distribution. This can be done for small samples as well as large. The one-sample or paired t method is used when we have data from the same sample or from matched samples. The method uses the differences between the paired observations and makes inferences about the mean difference in the population. The method requires that the differences must follow a Normal distribution and that mean difference is constant and so unrelated to the magnitude of the measurement. The two-sample or unpaired t test is used if we have means from two independent samples. It is also called the two-sample or independent t method. The two samples must be from Normal distributions with the same variance.

If data do not meet the assumptions, because the distribution is skew or the population variances cannot be assumed to be the same, we can often use a transformation such as the logarithm so that assumptions are met on the transformed scale. We then carry out t tests on the log transformed data.

We can use an F test to compare the variances of two samples from Normal distributions. An F test can also be used to compare the means of more than two groups in the one-way analysis of variance, with the same assumptions as the two-sample t test. If there is a significant difference overall, there are several multiple comparison tests available which allow comparisons to be made between pairs of groups. Analysis of variance can also be used when our interest is not in these particular groups but in a population of groups, for example when analysing repeated measurements on the same subjects. Here we estimate the variances between and within the groups.

When there are repeated measurements on the same subject, over time for example, summary statistics such as the area under the curve can be used and analyses done on these. When we have a trial randomized in clusters, summary statistics for each cluster, such as the mean or proportion, can be used as the variable in a two-sample t test.

QUESTIONS

10.1 Shortly after the grounding of the Braer oil tanker off the Shetland Isles, a study was conducted to ascertain whether the respiratory tracts of children were being affected by the crude oil vapour and droplet spray. Peak expiratory flow rate (PEFR) of 44 children aged 5–12 years was measured twice: 3 days after the shipwreck and 9–12 days after when the strong smell of oil had abated. Statistical analysis of the paired PEFRs (by Student's t test for difference of means for paired samples) showed no significant difference between the two sets of values (P = 0.502) (Crum 1993).

10.1.1 What is meant by no significant difference?

10.1.2 What is meant by a paired t test? What assumptions are involved and are they likely to be justified here?

10.1.3 What can we conclude about the effect of spillage on the respiratory function of children?

10.2 Questionnaires were sent to a random sample of 200 GPs in East Anglia, asking about their diagnosis and treatment of hypertension. Replies were received from 125 GPs. GPs were asked what was the minimum blood pressure they would regard as showing hypertension, and which was the minimum pressure at which they would begin treatment. The mean minimum diastolic pressure for treatment was 3.8 mm Hg higher for treatment than for diagnosis (95% CI 3.3 to 4.2 mm Hg). The paired t method was used in the analysis (Dickerson and Brown 1995).

What conditions do the data have to meet for the paired t method to be valid? Given the kind of response that these questions are likely to produce, is it likely that they were met in this study? What would the effect be if they were not?

ANSWERS

10.1.1 No significant difference is the result of a significance test comparing PEFR in children at two points in time after exposure. The null hypothesis is that there is no change in PEFR in the population from which the sample of children was drawn. The data was used to give a test statistic which has a t distribution if the null hypothesis is true. We then find the probability of data as or more extreme as that observed if the null hypothesis were true. If the probability is small, then we have good evidence against the null hypothesis. Conventionally, we use $P = 0.05$ as the cut-off. Here the probability must be > 0.05, therefore we conclude that the study failed to detect a difference. This does not necessarily mean that no difference exists since we cannot prove that the null hypothesis is true on the basis of a significance test (*Intro* §9.3).

10.1.2 The paired t test is used to test the null hypothesis as above. It is used here because we have two measurements on each subject at two points in time and we are interested in the differences within individuals. The t test can be used for small samples but requires that the differences follow a Normal distribution. This is likely to be true because PEFR follows a Normal distribution and the difference of two variables from Normal distributions will also follow a Normal distribution (*Intro* §10.2).

10.1.3 There is no evidence for a reduction in lung function in the children between 3 and 12 days after the spillage. However, we should not conclude that the spillage had no effect on lung function. There may be an effect which is too small to be statistically significant in a sample of this size. Alternatively, lung function may have already been reduced before the initial reading was taken and remained reduced (*Intro* §9.6).

10.2 For the paired t test to be valid the differences must be from a Normal distribution. They must also be unrelated to the magnitude of the measurement. We think it is unlikely that differences were from a Normal distribution here, because we think that most GPs would quote blood pressures to the nearest 5 or 10 mm Hg. Thus the differences would be 0, 5, 10, etc., and there would be only a few possible values. The effect would be to widen and bias the confidence interval. The effect would be quite small, because the sample is fairly large, greater than 100, and the large sample Normal approximation would apply (*Intro* §10.2).

QUESTIONS

10.3 The following table shows the serum cholesterol concentrations of 20 smokers and 20 non-smokers, matched for age and sex, recruited for a study of glucose response. Statistical analysis was by two-tailed, unpaired Student's t test (Facchini *et al.* 1992).

Cholesterol concentration, mean (SEM) in mmol/L

	Smokers	Non-smokers	t test
Total plasma	4.49 (0.19)	4.48 (0.17)	NS
Very low density lipoprotein (VLDL)	0.45 (0.06)	0.23 (0.04)	P < 0.005
Intermediate density lipoprotein (IDL)	0.18 (0.03)	0.22 (0.04)	NS
Low density lipoprotein (LDL)	2.72 (0.17)	2.53 (0.13)	NS
High density lipoprotein (HDL)	1.16 (0.05)	1.51 (0.08)	P < 0.005

10.3.1 What is meant by a 'two-tailed, unpaired Student's t test'?

10.3.2 What conditions must the data satisfy for these t tests to be valid? Are these likely to be satisfied here?

10.3.3 What extra information could be given in the table?

❶ 10.3.4 What aspect of the data has been ignored in the analysis?

10.4 In a randomized controlled trial carried out to evaluate the influence of pre-operative abstinence on post-operative outcome in alcohol misusers, 42 alcoholic patients admitted for elective colorectal surgery were allocated either to withdrawal from alcohol consumption for one month before operation (disulfiram controlled) or to carry on with their usual drinking (Tonnesen *et al.* 1999). Among others, glucose and adrenalin were measured at several times. The means at each time were as follows:

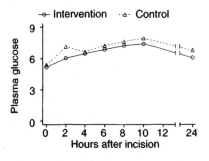 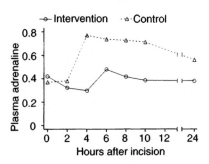

The authors analysed these as the area under the curve (AUC). The treatment difference was significant for adrenalin, not for glucose.

❶ 10.4.1 What is meant by 'area under the curve' and how can this be calculated?

❶ 10.4.2 What are the advantages of this approach compared to analysing each time point separately?

ANSWERS

10.3.1   The two-tailed, unpaired Student's t test is used to compare means from two independent samples. It tests the null hypothesis that the means are the same in the populations from which the samples are drawn against the alternative hypothesis of a difference in either direction. If the null hypothesis is true then the difference between means divided by the standard error of the difference follows the t distribution with 38 ($= 20 - 1 + 20 - 1$) degrees of freedom (*Intro* §9.5, 10.3).

10.3.2   The assumptions are that the cholesterol data are from Normal distributions with the same variance. In general serum concentrations are often positively skew with the variance increasing with the mean. Here, the standard errors are consistently bigger for the larger of the two means for each type of cholesterol. Since the sample size is equal for the smokers and non-smokers, the standard deviations must also increase with the means. Hence, the assumptions of the tests may not be met. However, with equal numbers in two groups the test is very robust, though some power may be lost (*Intro* §10.3, 10.5).

10.3.3   It would be useful to show the difference between the means and a 95% CI for that difference. In addition, the actual P value is more informative than 'NS'.

10.3.4   The analysis has ignored the matching for age and sex and has treated the groups as independent. A matched analysis, such as using a paired t test would take the structure of the data into account. If cholesterol is actually related to the matching variables age and sex, a paired test would remove some of the variation which is included in the standard error in the unpaired test. The paired test would be more powerful. If cholesterol were unrelated to the matching variables then a paired test would not be necessary. When the sample is very small, the loss of degrees of freedom may even make a paired test less powerful and so be counter-productive in these circumstances.

10.4.1   The AUC is a method for combining a series of measurements made at different times into a single observation. It takes into account the actual time intervals. These may vary, as in this example, where the last time interval (14 hours) is much longer than the others (all 2 hours). It is usually calculated by the trapezium method. For each time interval, the average of the measurements at the beginning and end is multiplied by the length of the interval. These are then added to give the AUC (*Intro* §10.7).

10.4.2   As the authors of this paper say, it reduces the number of tests and so reduces the risk of a spurious significant difference when the null hypothesis is true. It also uses all the information in a single test and so increases the power of the test, the chance of getting a significant difference when the null hypothesis is false (*Intro* §9.10, 10.7).

QUESTIONS

10.5   It was postulated that the increasing rate of hip fractures among elderly women may be related to women now having longer femoral necks than in previous generations. Fifty-two X-ray pictures of hips of elderly women taken in the 1950s were compared to 52 similar pictures taken in the 1990s. All the X-rays had been taken for routine diagnostic purposes with the same equipment in the same rheumatology unit (Reid *et al.* 1994). The following table appeared:

Mean (standard deviation) dimensions of proximal femur in
52 elderly white women in New Zealand in 1950s compared
with those of 52 in 1990s

Dimension (mm)	1950s	1990s	P value
Length of hip axis	124.0 (8.6)	130.5 (8.6)	0.0002
Length of femoral neck	79.4 (7.6)	84.9 (6.3)	0.0001
Width of femoral neck	38.1 (4.1)	38.6 (3.6)	0.49

10.5.1   What method could be used to calculate P in this study? What conditions, if any, do the data have to fulfil for the method to be valid? Are they likely to be fulfilled here?

10.5.2   From these P values, can we conclude that the length of femoral neck in elderly women has increased over time? Can we conclude that the width of femoral neck in elderly women has not increased over time?

10.6   In a study of factors predicting male fertility, conventional semen indices were measured in donors to an artificial insemination clinic. By evaluating the pregnancies that resulted, donors could be graded as to their fertility. No significant differences were found in semen indices for successful and unsuccessful donors.

Semen indices in most and least fertile donors

	Successful donors			Unsuccessful donors		
	No.	Mean	(SD)	No.	Mean	(SD)
Volume (ml)	17	3.14	(1.28)	19	2.91	(0.91)
Semen count (10^6/ml)	18	146.4	(95.7)	19	124.8	(81.8)
% motility	17	60.7	(9.7)	19	58.5	(12.8)
% abnormal morphology	13	22.8	(8.4)	16	20.3	(8.5)

All differences not significant, t test.

The study concluded that conventional semen analysis may be too insensitive an indicator of fertility potential (Paraskevaides *et al.* 1991).

10.6.1   Is there anything to suggest that the t test may not be valid?

10.6.2   What are the implications of this for the t test? What could be done about it?

10.6.3   Are the t tests important to the conclusions of the study?

ANSWERS

10.5.1 In this study we have means from two independent samples. Hence, we can use an unpaired t test to test the null hypothesis that the means are the same in the populations from which samples were drawn. This method would assume that the data are from Normal distributions, with the same variance. These variables are measurements of skeletal size which often follow a Normal distribution. The standard deviations are small in comparison with the means, providing no evidence of skewness. Alternatively we could use the large Normal comparison of two means. This would assume that the sample is large enough for the means to follow Normal distributions and for the standard deviations to be well estimated (*Intro* §10.3).

10.5.2 There is good evidence that the length of the femoral neck is different in the populations which these samples represent because the difference was statistically significant. To conclude that there is a change over time we must assume that the samples are truly representative of elderly white women in these two decades. There is no evidence that the width of the femoral neck is different in the populations which these samples represent because the difference was not significant. However, this does not mean that it has not changed. The sample may be too small to detect a change which has occurred. A confidence interval would be more informative. The difference is 0.5 with 95% confidence -1.0 to 2.0. The clinical implication is that elderly women in the 1990s had longer, but not thicker, femoral necks than similar women in the 1950s. Longer bones may be more likely to break and so this may explain any increase in fractured neck of femur.

10.6.1 It is not likely that semen count follows a Normal distribution. The standard deviation is more than half the mean, so mean minus 2 SD would be negative. We would expect 2.5% of observations to be below this if the distribution were Normal. This would imply negative values, which would be impossible.

10.6.2 The distribution must be positively skew, which means that the t test is not strictly speaking valid. The distribution could be made more symmetric by a log transformation (*Intro* §10.3).

10.6.3 The t tests are not important to the conclusions of the study. What we want to know is how good the semen index is at discriminating between fertile and infertile donors, not whether the mean level is different. The degree of overlap between the fertile and infertile populations is much more important. As the means and standard deviations suggest that there is much overlap, the conventional semen indices do not discriminate well. The sensitivity and specificity of the semen tests would be more useful (*Intro* §15.4).

QUESTIONS

10.7 In a study of renal function in chronic obstructive airways disease (COAD), urine samples were collected from 21 COAD patients and 18 healthy controls. Albumin excretion by COAD patients and controls is shown in the figure below. The difference was significant (t = 3.5, P < 0.001). All analyses were done using the logarithms of the observations (Wilkinson *et al.* 1993).

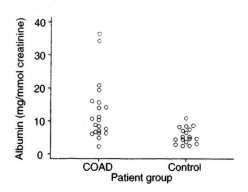

Why was the logarithmic transformation of the data used?

10.8 The effect of control of houseflies on the incidence of diarrhoea and shigellosis was evaluated at two military training camps. Fly traps were used at Base X for the 11 week training of a cohort of troops (early May to mid July), then used at Base Y for the training period of the next cohort (early August to mid October), no traps being used at Base X. The intervention was repeated during the next summer, the order of intervention being reversed. When fly control measures were used, clinic visits dropped by 42% (P = 0.146) for diarrhoeal diseases and by 85% for shigellosis (P = 0.015).

The analysis used the clinic morbidity rate for each base during each training session and averaged these to give an overall rate for the intervention and non-intervention bases. The two rates were arcsine transformed and then compared by Student's t test (one-tailed hypotheses) (Cohen *et al.* 1991).

10.8.1 Why might a transformation be necessary and what other transformations might have been considered?

10.8.2 Why did the authors not simply analyse the data by setting up a 2 × 2 table, traps used or not by infected or not, with each recruit providing a separate observation?

ANSWERS

10.7   From the figure we can see that the albumin data have skew distribu-
        tions, with a few observations much greater than the rest. The vari-
        ability is also much greater in the COAD patients where the mean is
        higher. Using a logarithmic scale (see figure below) stretches the bot-
        tom of the scale and compresses the top, making the distribution more
        like the Normal. The log transformation also makes the variances more
        uniform. The transformed data matches the assumptions of the t test
        more closely.

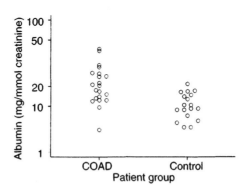

10.8.1 The variable is the proportion of the cohort who have disease. These are
        binomial proportions and hence have variance related to the magnitude
        of the proportion. The arcsine transformation has been used to stabilize
        the variance. Other transformations which could have been considered
        are logarithm, square root and reciprocal (*Intro* §10.4).

10.8.2 The intervention, using fly traps, was applied to the whole camp and
        hence to all individuals within that camp at the same time. Individuals
        within a camp are more similar to each other than to individuals in
        another camp and hence are not independent. To ignore this and to
        analyse at the level of the individual would underestimate the total
        variability. This could lead to spurious significant results as the standard
        error would be too small. Since the intervention was applied at the camp
        level, we must analyse the data at this level too (*Intro* §10.13).

QUESTIONS

10.9   In a study of factors related to coronary heart disease (CHD), the prevalence of arm movements was compared in 25 consecutive attenders at a
chest pain clinic who had CHD and 25 consecutive attenders at a non-
cardiac clinic. Patients were fitted with a goniometer, a device which
records movement. Movements were recorded during 10 min of the consultation. The function of the goniometer was not explained to the
patient until after the reading had been taken. The data are shown in
the graph below:

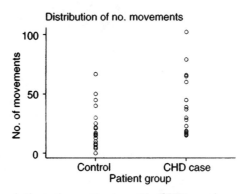

The study found that the patients with CHD made more arm movements than the controls. This difference was statistically significant
using one-way analysis of variance (P = 0.01) (Rennie 1997).

10.9.1   What is meant by one-way analysis of variance and what assumptions
about the data does it require?

10.9.2   Are these assumptions likely to be met here?

10.9.3   How could we use a transformation for these data? What problems
would be caused by the subject who had zero arm movements recorded?

10.9.4   What other equivalent method could have been used to give the P value?

ANSWERS

10.9.1   Analysis of variance is a statistical technique used when we wish to compare the means of several groups. Analysis of variance uses the data from all of the groups to estimate the standard error and so is more powerful than doing t tests on pairs of groups. The method requires that the data come from a Normal distribution and that the variance is the same in all of the groups.

10.9.2   Inspection of the data redrawn from the original paper shows that the data are positively skew and the variance is slightly higher in the group with the higher mean (CHD cases). This suggests that the data should be transformed prior to analysis.

10.9.3   The figure below shows the data after logarithmic and square root transformation. The observation which is zero causes a problem for log transformation, as zero has no logarithm. We have set this to the log of half the next largest observation (4), which is a bit arbitrary but better than making it a missing value. Another possibility would be to add a small number, such as one, before transforming. The log transformation corrects the skewness. However, the variance in the CHD cases is now less than in the controls so the transformation has over-corrected. A square root transformation looks better. The variable is a count of the number movements in a fixed time and therefore might be expected to have a Poisson distribution. The square root transformation is the correct variance-stabilizing and Normalizing transformation for the Poisson, so this is plausible.

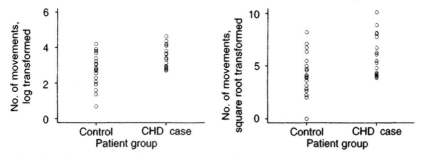

The P value from the analysis of variance using the square root transformation is just smaller than that for the log transformation (untransformed: $P = 0.0134$, log: $P = 0.0071$, square root: $P = 0.0066$). Making the data fit the assumptions of the method better usually reduces the P value.

10.9.4   When there are only two groups to compare, one-way analysis of variance is exactly equivalent to a two-sample t test, making the same assumptions about the data and giving the same P value.

11
Regression and correlation

Regression and correlation are used to investigate relationships between two continuous variables. Regression is used to predict one variable, Y, from the other, X. The regression equation is $Y = a + bX$. Here b is the slope of the regression line, the estimated change in Y per unit increase in X, and a is the intercept, the predicted value of Y when $X = 0$. The line is found by the method of least squares. We often test the null hypothesis that the slope is zero in the population, or find a CI for the slope. The method requires that the outcome variable, Y, should have deviations from the line which follow a Normal distribution for any given value of X, with uniform variance along the line.

The correlation coefficient, r, measures the strength of the linear relationship between two continuous variables. It lies between -1 and $+1$, 0 for no relationship. A positive correlation shows that Y tends to be high when X is high. A negative correlation shows that Y tends to be low when X is high. We often test the null hypothesis that the correlation coefficient is zero in the population. For this test at least one of the variables must be from a Normal distribution. The tests of the null hypothesis of no linear relationship using regression and correlation are numerically identical. We can calculate a confidence interval for the correlation coefficient, but both variables must follow Normal distributions for this.

If data do not meet the assumptions because the distribution is positively skew or the variances are not uniform we can often use a transformation such as the logarithm and carry out regression or correlation on the transformed data.

When using these techniques, observations should be independent. We should not have several pairs of observations from each subject, for example.

The intraclass correlation coefficient (ICC) is used when the same variable is measured more than once on the same subject, for example in the study of measurement error. In calculating ICCs, the order in which measurements were made is ignored.

QUESTIONS

11.1   In a study of blood pressure during pregnancy and fetal growth, 209
healthy women having their first pregnancy had 24 hour blood pressure
readings taken in mid-pregnancy. The size of the baby was recorded
at birth. The abstract included the following: 'It was found that a
5 mm Hg increase in mean 24 hour diastolic blood pressure at 28 weeks'
gestation was associated with a 68 g (95% CI 3 to 132) decrease in birth
weight ... Maternal mean 24 hour diastolic blood pressure at 28 weeks'
gestation was also inversely associated with the infant's ponderal index
(weight/height^3) at birth ... (P = 0.06).' (Churchill and Beevers 1997).
(NB: weight/height^3 is the usual ponderal index for infants, rather than
weight/height^2 as is used for adults and older children.)

11.1.1   What method would be used to calculate the 68 g per 5 mm Hg?

11.1.2   What assumptions would the method require?

11.1.3   What is meant by 'increase' and 'decrease' here? Do they mean that
when a woman's blood pressure went down her baby's weight went up?

11.2   In a study of neuron loss and ageing, brains were studied from a group
of 38 subjects, ages 13–101 years, who had died without any history of
long-term illness or dementia. Neurons were counted in a part of the
brain called the hippocampus. This was done in several sections of each
region of the hippocampus and hence an estimate of the total number
of neurons in the region was made. Counting was done without the
investigator being aware of the age of the subject (West *et al.* 1994).
Some of the results were as follows:

Relationship of total number of neurons to age, normal subjects		
Hippocampus sub-division	Slope of neurons versus age (number/year)	P
Dentate granule cell layer	−54 000	0.17
Dentate hilus	−9 000	0.012
Pyramidal cell layer CA3-2	−6 000	0.18
Pyramidal cell layer CA1	−29 000	0.26
Subiculum	−36 000	0.001 3

11.2.1   What is meant by slope of neurons versus age? Why are the slopes
negative?

11.2.2   Why were data collected without the observer being aware of the age of
the subject?

ANSWERS

11.1.1 Sixty-eight grams per 5 mm Hg is calculated using simple linear regression. This method estimates the nature of the relationship between two continuous variables, here mean 24-hour diastolic blood pressure and infant birthweight. The quantity given comes directly from the slope of the line. The method works by calculating the line of best fit through the data using the principle of least squares (*Intro* §11.2, 11.3).

11.1.2 This method would require that birthweight followed a Normal distribution with the same variance for any given values of mean 24-hour diastolic blood pressure (*Intro* §11.3).

11.1.3 In this study blood pressure at 28 weeks is related to birthweight, a quantity which is measured once, at birth. This analysis is not investigating how changes in blood pressure within individuals might affect the growth of the baby. The increase in birthweight associated with a decrease in blood pressure therefore refers to the mean effect rather than an effect for an individual. The difference in mean birthweight between two groups of women whose mean blood pressure differ by 5 mm Hg would therefore be 68 g, with the direction of the difference being that women with lower mean blood pressure have greater mean birthweight.

11.2.1 The slope is the estimated change in neurons per year of age. It is the slope of the regression line. The slopes are negative because the number of neurons decreases with increasing age (*Intro* §11.2).

11.2.2 The investigator might expect that older people would have fewer neurons than young people. If the investigator knew the age, he/she might expect a small number of neurons in old subjects, and so count less carefully. The number of neurons might be underestimated. The slope would then be biased downwards (*Intro* §2.9).

QUESTIONS

11.3   A general practice based study sought to find out if people's ears increase in size as they get older. Two hundred and six patients were studied with ear size being assessed by the length of the left external ear from the top to the lowest part. Measurements were made simply, using a transparent plastic ruler. The relation between the patient's age and ear length (see graph below) was examined by calculating a regression equation:

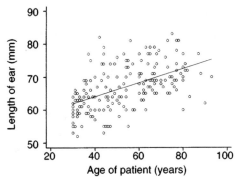

Mean age of patient was 53.75 years (range 30–93) and mean ear length was 67.5 mm (range 52.0–84.0 mm). The linear regression equation was ear length = 55.9 + 0.22 × age with a 95% CI for the b coefficient being 0.17 to 0.27. The author concluded that 'It seems therefore that as we get older our ears get bigger (on average by 0.22 mm a year)' (Heathcote 1995).

11.3.1   Is the distribution of ear size skew or symmetrical and why?

11.3.2   Is the distribution of age skew or symmetrical and why?

11.3.3   What are the interpretations of the numbers 55.9 and 0.22 in the regression equation?

11.3.4   Are the assumptions about the data are required for the regression analysis satisfied here?

11.3.5   What are the conclusions and are they justified by the data?

11.3.6   What further investigations could be done?

ANSWERS

11.3.1   It appears to be symmetrical. The mean (67.5) is almost exactly in the middle of the range (52.0–84.0), i.e. (52.0+84.0)/2 = 68.0. The figure also suggests this (*Intro* §4.4).

11.3.2   In this study age is positively skew. The mean is closer to the minimum than to the maximum.

11.3.3   The regression line shows the estimated mean ear size for given age. The line has slope 0.22, i.e. mean ear size increases by 0.22 mm for each year of age. When age is zero, the line would cross the vertical axis at 55.9. This does not mean that babies have ears of this size, because we would be extrapolating beyond the data. We cannot do this because we cannot assume that the straight line relationship will also be valid for children (*Intro* §11.2).

11.3.4   We assume that the deviations from the regression line follow a Normal distribution and have uniform variation along the line. The second assumption looks very reasonable from the figure. The spread of the data about the line is very similar all the way along. It is difficult to tell about the Normal distribution. There appears to be some deviation from linearity, as the points tend to be below the line at each end. This may be because the older people will tend to be women, who are smaller than men (*Intro* §11.3).

11.3.5   This is a cross-sectional not a longitudinal study, and the uncertainty in the estimate should be included. Strictly speaking, the conclusions should read 'It seems therefore that older people have bigger ears (on average by between 0.17 and 0.27 mm per year of age)'. It could be that the ears of different birth cohorts differ. After all, different birth cohorts have different mean heights at the same age. (Personally, we think that the author's interpretation is correct, but we cannot draw this conclusion from these data alone.)

11.3.6   For these data, it would be interesting to look at men and women separately. Is it old men who have big ears, or old people? Ideally, we would like to follow people over time, if not from cradle to grave at least for several years, to see whether this is a phenomenon of individual growth or of differences between generations.

QUESTIONS

11.4   The birthweights of 1 333 fifty-year-old Swedish men were traced
through birth records. Adult height and birthweight were significantly
correlated ($r = 0.22$, P < 0.001) (Leon *et al.* 1996).

11.4.1   What is meant by 'correlated' and '$r = 0.22$'?

11.4.2   What assumptions are required for the calculation of the P value?

11.4.3   What can we conclude about the relationship between adult height and
birthweight?

11.5   A survey of radon concentration in houses in a small town was used
to investigate the relationship between mutant frequency in peripheral
lymphocytes, and domestic radon concentration. Non-smoking subjects
were selected from a GP list, non-randomly, so as to give a wide range
of radon exposures. The results are shown in the figure. The relationship was statistically significant (t = 3.47, d.f. = 17, P < 0.01) (Bridges
et al. 1991).

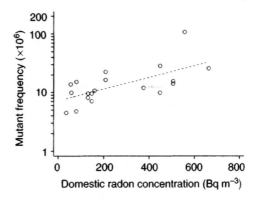

11.5.1   What kind of scale is used on the vertical axis?

❗ 11.5.2   What was done to the mutant frequency before the line was estimated?

❗ 11.5.3   Why were the author correct not to calculate and present a correlation
coefficient using the original variables?

ANSWERS

11.4.1 Two variables are correlated if when one has high values, the other has high values and when one has low values, the other has low values, or if when one has high values the other has low values and when one has low values, the other has high values. r is the correlation coefficient which measures the strength of the linear relationship between two continuous variables. It lies between -1 and $+1$ with 0 showing no relationship. $r = 0.22$ is a positive correlation, showing that adult height tends to be greater for subjects with high birthweight but the relationship is weak and would be hard to see on a scatter diagram (*Intro* §11.9).

11.4.2 One of the two variables must follow a Normal distribution for the P value to be valid.

11.4.3 In the population which these subjects represent, adult height is related to birthweight, but the relationship is weak. Tall men tend to have been heavier at birth. We cannot conclude from these data, however, that the relationship is causal.

11.5.1 This is a logarithmic scale (*Intro* §5.9).

11.5.2 The mutant frequency was log transformed for the analysis. The regression line has been calculated using the transformed data. Transformation back to the original scale would give an exponential curve rather than a straight line. Using a log scale on the graph restores this to a straight line.

11.5.3 The sample is non-random and so would not represent the population. The radon exposures have been chosen to include extreme observations. This would inflate the value of the correlation coefficient and it would not estimate anything useful.

QUESTIONS

11.6 Notifications of tuberculosis and several indicators of poverty were recorded in the 33 electoral wards of Liverpool. The tuberculosis notification rate was correlated with the percentage of children in the electoral ward who received free school meals ($r = 0.44$, $P < 0.01$) (Spence *et al.* 1993). A figure similar to that below was presented:

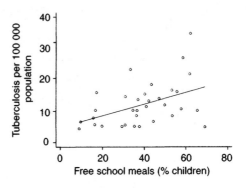

11.6.1 What kind of study is this?

11.6.2 How could the statistical analysis be improved?

11.6.3 The authors did not conclude that school meals cause tuberculosis. Why were they correct and what conclusions would you draw?

11.7 A graph similar to the following appeared in a study of epilepsy and psychological function. Scores on two psychological tests are plotted against age for 63 epileptic patients, with regression lines. For 125 controls, the regression lines of score on age are given, but not the individual data points (Helmstaedter and Elger 1999).

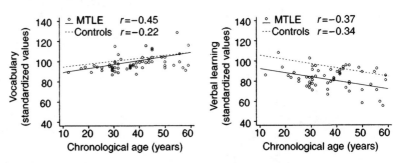

11.7.1 Assuming the data are correct, what are the obvious misprints on this graph?

11.7.2 What can we conclude about the differences in psychological test performance between epileptics and controls?

ANSWERS

11.6.1   This is an ecological study where the observations are the percentage of children having free school meals and the tuberculosis rate in 33 electoral wards.

11.6.2   Tuberculosis rate is clearly skew and the variability increases as we move from left to right. A log transformation helps (see figure below), though in this case the correlation coefficient and P value change very little.

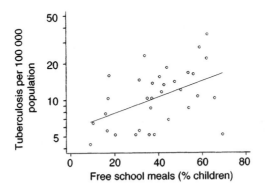

11.6.3   This is an observational study and so we cannot assume that an association implies causation. In addition this is an ecological study, not a study of individuals. It is not necessarily the children eating school meals who get tuberculosis. To draw a causal conclusion would be an example of the ecological fallacy. In this study free school meals has been used as a proxy measure for social deprivation. All that we can conclude is that wards which have a high proportion of children receiving free school meals tend to have a high notification rate for tuberculosis. With $r = 0.44$, the relationship is not very strong (*Intro* §3.10).

11.7.1   The correlation coefficients for vocabulary should be positive. Following a letter from ourselves, the following correction was printed *Lancet* (2000): '... the correlation coefficients for vocabulary scores in the figure should be $r = 0.45$ for patients with mesial temporal-lobe epilepsy (MTLE) and $r = 0.22$ for controls ...'.

11.7.2   There is no evidence of any difference in vocabulary. The regression lines are virtually identical, so the mean vocabulary score at any age is the same for epileptics and controls. For verbal learning ability, the lines are parallel but separated by a vertical distance of more than 10 points. There is no evidence that epileptics lose verbal learning ability faster than controls, but their level is lower at each age. These were the conclusions of the authors (Helmstaedter and Elger 1999).

QUESTIONS

11.8   In a study of acute myeloid leukaemia (AML) and domestic radiation, incidence of disease was related to mean indoor radon concentration estimate (Bequerels per cubic metre) for 23 geographical areas. Indoor radiation was estimated by placing meters in a small sample of homes in each area (Lucie 1989).

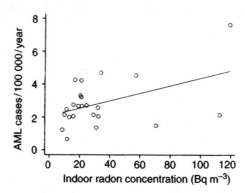

The author reported the correlation coefficient (0.45) to be significant (P < 0.05).

11.8.1   What kind of study is this?

11.8.2   What does the correlation coefficient tell us in this study?

11.8.3   Do the assumptions for regression and correlation appear to be met in the figure? What other graphs might be drawn to test them?

11.8.4   What alternative analysis could be done if the assumptions are not met?

11.8.5   What is the main difficulty arising from the design of this study?

ANSWERS

11.8.1 This is an ecological study, where the analysis is at the level of a geo-
        graphical area.

11.8.2 $r = 0.45$ is a positive correlation of moderate size and tells us that
        indoor radiation concentration and AML are related in this sample, but
        not closely.

11.8.3 For the test of the correlation coefficient, at least one of the variables
        should follow a Normal distribution. Inspection of the diagram suggest
        that both variables are skew. We could investigate this further by his-
        tograms or Normal plots of the two variables. For the regression, we
        must assume that the residuals, observed AML values minus the value
        predicted by regression, follow a Normal distribution and have the same
        variance all the way along the line. We can calculate the residuals and
        construct a Normal plot, and we can plot them against the radon. Here
        the residuals appear to follow a Normal distribution reasonably, but
        they are much more variable at the high radon end than for low radon.

11.8.4 We can try a logarithmic transformation to see whether the data fit the
        requirements better afterwards, which it appears that they do:

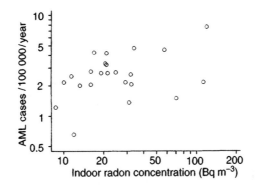

        For the log data, the correlation coefficient becomes non-significant,
        $r = 0.39$, P $= 0.07$. Alternatively, we could use rank correlation (*Intro*
        §12.4, 12.5).

11.8.5 The problem is, as is usually the case with ecological studies, that the
        people whose homes were measured are not actually those who have
        AML. We can only say that in areas where the radiation in homes is
        high, there may be a higher rate of AML. The relationship is indirect
        and there may be many possible explanations apart from the obvious
        causal one.

QUESTIONS

11.8.6 What further studies could be done to investigate the theory that domestic radiation increases the risk of AML?

11.9 In a randomized double-blind, placebo-controlled trial of human recombinant growth hormone (rhGH) in patients with chronic heart failure, 50 patients were allocated to treatment or placebo. The figure below shows the relationship between changes in serum IGF-1 (a growth factor) and changes in left-ventricular mass by treatment group. The authors reported that 'by linear regression analysis a significant relation was found between changes in serum IGF-1 concentrations and left-ventricular mass for all patients ($r = 0.55$, P $= 0.0001$) but this relation was less evident when the two groups were analysed separately (rhGH $r = 0.28$, P $= 0.19$; placebo $r = 0.36$, P $= 0.08$)' (Osterziel *et al.* 1998):

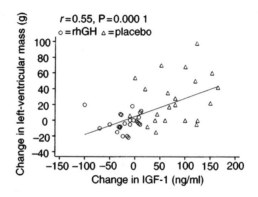

Suggest why the relation between changes in IGF-1 and changes in left-ventricular mass as shown in the graph was 'less evident when the two groups were analysed separately'.

11.10 Female twins, 130 identical and 120 non-identical pairs, were screened radiologically for osteoarthritis. The intraclass correlation of the total radiographic osteoarthritis score in identical pairs was 0.64 (SE 0.05) compared with 0.38 (0.08) in non-identical pairs (Spector *et al.* 1996).

11.10.1 What is meant by 'intraclass correlation'? Why was this correlation coefficient used here?

11.10.2 What can we conclude about the relative contribution of genetic and environmental factors to osteoarthritis?

ANSWERS

11.8.6   Further studies include a case–control study, comparing radiation in the homes of AML cases and controls without AML, or a cohort study, measuring radiation in a very large number of homes and observing any subsequent cases of AML.

11.9   In this study we have 2 separate groups, rhGH and placebo, in which the distributions of IGF-1 hardly overlap. It appears that the rhGH treatment has increased both IGF-1 and left-ventricular mass. Putting the two groups together in this way increases the range of the data and so increases the size of the correlation. It also produces a mixture of two populations, treated and untreated. The relationship between IGF and mass at the individual level is confused with that at the group level, an effect similar to that produced by combining multiple observations from each subject (*Intro* §11.12). It is, therefore, misleading to calculate a correlation coefficient for the combined data. These data could be analysed together using a multiple regression approach (*Intro* §17.1).

11.10.1   The usual product moment correlation coefficient has two variables, usually denoted by X and Y. Sometimes it is not obvious which of a pair of observations is X and which Y, for example if the observations are measurements made on a pair of twins. Which twin is X and which is Y? The ICC is the average correlation which we would get if we took all possible orderings of the twin pairs. As the choice of twins to be X and Y is arbitrary, the ICC is the appropriate correlation coefficient (*Intro* §11.13).

11.10.2   Identical twins share the same genes and usually the same early environment. Non-identical twins of the same sex share only 50% of their genes and usually share the same childhood environment. Thus if identical twins are more similar in some characteristic than non-identical twins, this provides evidence that there is a genetic influence on that characteristic. The authors of this study concluded that 'These results demonstrate ... a clear genetic effect for radiographic osteoarthritis of the hand and knee in women'.

QUESTIONS

11.11 A sample of 15 283 subjects drawn from GP lists completed questionnaires to measure fatigue and psychological morbidity. The fatigue scale
consisted of 11 questions and each was scored 0 or 1 to give a total score
between 0 and 11. Psychological morbidity was measured by the general
health questionnaire (GHQ), consisting of 12 questions scored similarly
to give a total score between 0 and 12. The authors reported that scores
on the fatigue and GHQs were moderately correlated ($r = 0.62$, 95%
CI 0.61 to 0.63) with a linear trend between fatigue score and mean
GHQ score (Pawlikowska *et al.* 1994). A graph similar to the following
was presented, showing the mean and 95% CI for GHQ score according
to fatigue score:

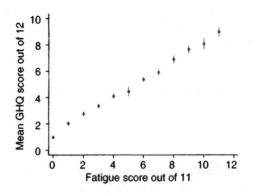

❗➕ 11.11.1 Why does this graph give an exaggerated idea of the strength of the
relationship?

❗ 11.11.2 How might a graph giving a realistic impression of the strength of the
relationship be presented?

The subjects were drawn from five general practice lists: a health centre
in south London, an inner city London practice, a practice located on the
Surrey–Hampshire border, a practice in an urban area of a south coast
port, and a practice in a Somerset village. Questionnaires were sent to
all patients aged 18–45 years registered with these selected practices.
No account appears to have been taken of this sample structure in the
analysis.

➕ 11.11.3 What kind of sampling is this?

❗➕ 11.11.4 How might the sample structure produce misleading results in the analysis?

➕ 11.11.5 How might the sample structure be allowed for in the analysis?

ANSWERS

11.11.1 For each level of fatigue score, the mean and its 95% CI was plotted. Because the sample was very large, the confidence intervals are very narrow. The graph gives no idea of the variation about the line which could be drawn through the group means. Using confidence intervals like this makes the relationship look very close, but as the authors say the correlation coefficient of 0.62 is only moderate.

11.11.2 A simple scatter diagram will not work, because there are 15 000 points. One possibility would be to show the mean and a 95% range for GHQ for each fatigue level, i.e. a line from the 2.5 percentile to the 97.5 percentile. Another possibility would be to draw a box and whisker plot of GHQ for each fatigue level. There are insufficient data in the paper for us to guess what these graphs might look like.

11.11.3 This is a cluster sample, the five practices being the clusters (*Intro* §3.4).

11.11.4 It is quite possible that people living in socially deprived areas suffer more psychological morbidity and more fatigue than those living in rural areas. Thus a relationship might be generated which is due to area rather than to a relationship at the level of individual (*Intro* §11.12). We do not know that this is the case, of course, only that it might be and should be dealt with in the analysis.

11.11.5 The best way would be to carry out a multiple regression analysis with GHQ as the outcome variable and fatigue score and practice as predictors. We could use this to estimate a correlation within the practice (*Intro* §17.1, Bland and Altman 1995).

12
Methods based on rank order

The questions in this chapter cover material which would usually be found only in advanced courses.

Methods based on rank order are non-parametric, meaning that we do not assume that the data come from a distribution, such as the Normal, the parameters of which must be estimated from the data. Non-parametric methods require fewer assumptions about the data than do methods which require the assumption that data come from a particular family of distributions, but are less powerful when the assumptions are met. To provide confidence intervals, most rank-based methods require very strong assumptions about the data. Rank methods are primarily tests of significance.

Most of these methods require only that the data be ordinal, i.e. that we can arrange the observations in ascending order. The actual observed values are not used. The Wilcoxon signed-rank matched-pairs test requires interval data, where we can subtract one observation from another.

The Mann–Whitney U test (or its alternative formulation, the Wilcoxon two-sample test) is used to compare two independent groups. The sign test and the Wilcoxon signed-rank matched-pairs test are used to test for changes in a single sample or to compare matched samples.

Spearman's rank correlation coefficient, ρ or rho, and Kendall's rank correlation coefficient, τ or tau, are used to test the relationship between two variables which need only be on ordinal scales of measurement. The Kendall method deals with ties better and has several variants for dealing with these.

QUESTIONS

12.1   A group of researchers observed that baby boys had higher pain scores
following vaccination than baby girls. They hypothesized that this
might be partly related to previous experience with acute pain such
as circumcision. They therefore sought to investigate *post hoc* whether
male neonatal circumcision is associated with a greater pain response to
routine vaccination at 4 or 6 months. They scored pain response after
vaccination with *Haemophilus influenzae* type B (HIB) ($n = 18$). An
independent observer rated the pain responses for each baby on a scale
from 0 (no pain) to 10 (worst pain) as shown in the figure:

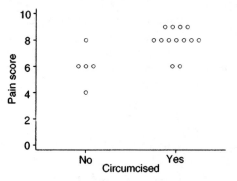

After HIB, pain score was significantly higher in boys who had previ-
ously been circumcised (Mann–Whitney U test, P = 0.01) (Taddio *et al.*
1995).

12.1.1   What is the Mann–Whitney U test?

12.1.2   What feature of the data makes the authors use the Mann–Whitney U
test here? Is it necessary here?

12.1.3   What are the disadvantages of this method compared to methods based
on the Normal distribution?

ANSWERS

12.1.1   This is a hypothesis test which compares the distribution of pain in two independent groups, here baby boys who have and who have not been circumcised. The test is based on the ranks of the data rather than on the data values themselves. It is a non-parametric analogue of the two-sample t test.

12.1.2   The data here are discrete, rather than continuous, varying between 0 and 10. Thus the data cannot follow a Normal distribution. The two-sample t test would therefore only be approximate and the Mann–Whitney U test is used since it only requires the data to be ordinal.

12.1.3   The main disadvantage of the Mann–Whitney U test is that it is a significance test and gives a P value but does not give a simple estimate and confidence interval for the difference between the groups. The test statistic U can be used to derive the probability that a randomly chosen observation from one population will exceed a randomly chosen observation from the other population. However, this is not straightforward to interpret. Methods based on the Normal distribution such as the t test would give an estimate of the difference and confidence interval in addition to the P value. The t test is fairly robust to grouping and so might have been used here thus giving a mean difference (2.0) and 95% CI (0.8 to 3.2).

QUESTIONS

12.2 The volume of the spleen was measured by CT scan in 25 patients with acute pancreatitis. The initial measurement was made within 3 days of onset, the first follow-up between 4 and 30 days, and the second follow-up between 31 and 100 days. Five patients had measurements available before onset. The percentage increases in spleen size over the initial measurement are shown in the figure:

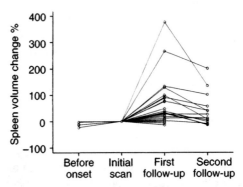

The volume of the spleen increased significantly between the initial scan and the first follow-up ($P < 0.0001$). At the second follow-up, there was a significant decline from the first follow-up ($P < 0.002$). The tests were done using the Wilcoxon signed-rank test (Tsushima *et al.* 1999).

➕ 12.2.1 What is the Wilcoxon signed-rank test and for what type of data is it suitable?

➕ 12.2.2 Why is the Wilcoxon signed-rank test appropriate for these data?

➕ 12.2.3 We could analyse these data by the sign test. What would be the advantages and disadvantages compared to the Wilcoxon signed-rank test?

➕ 12.2.4 We could analyse these data by the paired t test. What would be the advantages and disadvantages compared to the Wilcoxon signed-rank test?

❗➕ 12.2.5 Why could the Wilcoxon signed-rank test not be used to test changes from the scans made before the onset of the disease?

ANSWERS

12.2.1 This is the non-parametric analogue of the paired t test. The test is based on the ranks of the data rather than on the data values themselves. It can be used when we have matched interval level data on a single group of individuals (*Intro* §12.3).

12.2.2 The data are interval level, as they are based on physical measurements. The distributions of the increases are clearly very skew, so a paired t test would not be appropriate (*Intro* §12.3).

12.2.3 The advantage would be that we would not have to assume the data were interval. In this example, the data are clearly on an interval scale, so this is unimportant. The disadvantage would be that the power would be less. We get P = 0.0002 and P = 0.0001, respectively, so the conclusions would be the same (*Intro* §9.2).

12.2.4 The advantage would be that we would get a confidence interval and that if the differences were from a Normal distribution we would have more power. The disadvantage would be that we need the differences to be from a Normal distribution. From the graph, they are clearly positively skew. We might try a log transformation. We cannot do this on the percentage increases, as some of them are negative, but we can do it on the spleen volumes as a percentage of the initial CT measurement, obtained by adding 100 to all the increases. To our surprise, it did not work:

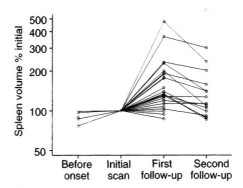

The percentage volumes shown on a logarithmic scale are clearly still positively skew. The Wilcoxon signed-rank test seems to be the best available analysis for these data (*Intro* §10.2).

12.2.5 The Wilcoxon signed-rank test cannot give a significant two-sided test unless there are at least six observations. All possible orderings have probablities greater than 0.025. There were only five measurements made before disease onset (*Intro* §12.3).

QUESTIONS

12.3   It is often necessary to take blood from newborn babies, which causes
them pain. Carbajal *et al.* (1999) randomly allocated 150 newborns
undergoing venepuncture to one of six treatment groups: no treatment;
placebo (2 ml sterile water); 2 ml 30% glucose; 2 ml 30% sucrose; a pacifier (or dummy); and 2 ml 30% sucrose followed by a pacifier. Each
venepuncture was observed by an assessor, who rated the baby's pain
on the DAN scale (Douleur Aiguë du Nouveau-ne). This rates pain on
a scale from 0 (no pain) to 10 (Carbajal *et al.* 1997). DAN is based on
observation of the baby's facial expression, limb movement, and vocal
expression.

12.3.1   This trial gives a new meaning to 'dummy treatment'. What is the
purpose of the placebo and to what extent is the trial blind?

The results are shown in the following figure:

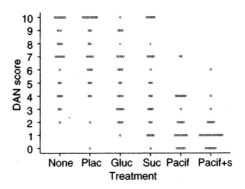

The results were presented as median (interquartile range) pain scores
during venepuncture. These were 7 (5–10) for no treatment; 7 (6–10)
for placebo; 5 (3–7) for 30% glucose; 5 (2–8) for 30% sucrose; 2 (1–4)
for pacifier; and 1 (1–2) for 30% sucrose plus pacifier.

12.3.2   Why might the authors have chosen to present their results in this way,
rather than as means and standard deviations? Are there any disadvantages for these data?

✚ 12.3.3   The Mann–Whitney U test was used to compare pairs of treatment
groups. What is the advantage of a rank-based method here?

✚ 12.3.4   What rank-based method could be used to test the null hypothesis that
there was no difference between any of the treatments?

ANSWERS

12.3.1   The placebo is to blind the observer, not the baby. This can only be partially successful, as the observer can only be blinded between the placebo and the sucrose and glucose solutions.

12.3.2   They do not actually quote the interquartile range, which is the difference between the third and first quartiles, but the quartiles themselves. This approach is sometimes adopted for skew data, although there is no reason why means and standard deviations should not be calculated when the distribution is skew. More seriously, the scale may not be interval, i.e. we cannot subtract on it, and therefore we cannot estimate a standard deviation. The disadvantage is that the data can take only a few integer values. The medians will all be integers, making it a rather crude summary statistic.

12.3.3   Inspection of the figure shows that the distribution is positively skew for some groups and negatively skew for others. Thus, the data do not follow a Normal distribution and would be difficult to transform to the Normal. The variances also vary between the groups. These problems arise because the scale is limited at 0 and 10 and there are several observations at each limit. Also, if we do not want to treat the scale as interval a rank method is appropriate.

12.3.4   The Kruskal–Wallis test is a method based on rank order that can be used to test the null hypothesis that several groups come from the same population. It is a generalization of the Mann–Whitney U test to several groups in the same way that one-way analysis of variance is a generalization of the two-sample t test. Here we get $P = 0.0001$. Hence, we can conclude that there are clear differences in DAN score between the treatments.

QUESTIONS

As multiple pairwise comparisons were made, the authors decided to consider P values less than 0.01 as significant. The P values for comparisons of 30% glucose, 30% sucrose, pacifier, and 30% sucrose plus pacifier versus placebo were 0.005, 0.01, < 0.0001, and < 0.0001, respectively. P values for comparisons of 30% glucose, 30% sucrose, and 30% sucrose plus pacifier versus pacifier were 0.0001, 0.001, and 0.06, respectively.

12.3.5 Why was a lower critical P value than usual adopted? Was the value chosen appropriate?

Differences between group median pain scores for these comparisons were 2 (95% CI 1 to 4), 2 (0 to 4), 5 (4 to 7), and 6 (5 to 8), respectively. Differences between group medians for 30% glucose, 30% sucrose, and 30% sucrose plus pacifier versus pacifier were 3 (2 to 5), 3 (1 to 5), and 1 (0 to 2), respectively.

12.3.6 What assumptions about the data are required for these Mann–Whitney-based confidence intervals? Are they met?

12.4 Pettersson *et al.* (1999) studied patients on entry to an 'Asthma School', where they were taught about their disease and its management, and 12 months later. They also compared the patients on entry to a national reference group drawn from the general Swedish population. They compared these groups using a quality of life measurement, the Sickness Impact Profile (SIP). The results for the psychosocial dimension of the SIP were:

	n	Mean	SD	Median	Range
Before Asthma School	32	4.1	8.1	0.0	0.0–33.1
12 months after Asthma School	32	4.3	7.4	0.0	0.0–24.8
Swedish national reference group	145	1.6	4.2	0.0	0.0–28.9

The authors compared the psychosocial dimension of the SIP before and after the Asthma School using a sign test, reported as 'n.s.'. They compared the patients before the Asthma School to the reference sample using a two-sample t test, reporting $P < 0.05$.

12.4.1 What can we conclude about the shape of the distribution of the psychosocial dimension of the SIP? What three features of the data support this?

12.4.2 Was the sign test an appropriate test?

ANSWERS

12.3.5 When null hypotheses are true, each test we do has probability 1/20 of giving a P value less than 0.05. When we do many tests, the chance of a spurious significant difference increases. If we were to do 20 independent tests we would expect 1. Here, we have the results of 7 tests presented, though 15 could have been done. Were 15 independent tests to be done the probability of a spurious significant difference would be $1 - 0.95^{15} = 0.54$. These tests are not independent, because the same six groups are involved in all of them, so this figure is only approximate. One approach is to ignore the multiple tests and interpret each comparison separately. Another, adopted here, is to lower the critical P value, so that if the null hypotheses are true, the chance of a spurious P value less than the critical value is reduced. Lowering the critical value reduces the power of the study, of course. For a critical value of 0.01, the probability that 15 independent tests will give at least one significant P value is $1 - 0.99^{15} = 0.14$. This seems a reasonable compromise between type I and type II errors. Another approach would be to use the Bonferroni correction, multiplying each P value by the number of tests. This would provide a valid (but not very powerful) test of the null hypothesis that all six groups come from the same population (i.e. that there are no treatment differences). It seems unnecessary here, as the comparisons between individual treatments are the main interest.

12.3.6 The Mann–Whitney confidence interval method assumes that the two distributions have exactly the same shape and differ in location (mean or median) only (Campbell and Gardner 1989). Clearly this is not true, as the distributions for some groups are negatively skew (no treatment, placebo) and for others are positively skew (pacifier, pacifier plus sucrose). Also, the variability is less for pacifier and for pacifier plus sucrose than for the other treatments. If the distributions differ only in location, their variances must be the same. The method also assumes that the scale of measurement is interval, because it requires calculating differences between observations in the two groups. The Mann–Whitney tests of significance are valid, but the confidence intervals are not. A two-sample t method would not be valid either, of course, so both approaches here would give an approximation only.

12.4.1 The distribution is positively skew. The median is considerably less than the mean, the standard deviation is greater than the mean, the median is equal to the lower limit of the range. Most of the observations must be zero.

12.4.2 The sign test is appropriate here, because the distribution of differences will not be Normal. Many of them will be zero.

QUESTIONS

12.4.3   How could the results of the sign test have been better reported?

12.4.4   What conditions should data meet for a two-sample t test to be valid? Do the data meet these conditions?

12.4.5   What alternative test could have been used to compare the Asthma School patients with the reference sample?

12.5   A Scottish study investigated the relation between grommet insertion operations and tonsillectomy rates (Bisset and Russell 1994). Health boards with high grommet insertion rates were more likely to have low tonsillectomy rates (Spearman's rank correlation $= -0.59$; 95% CI -0.87 to -0.03). The following graph has been drawn from the data presented in the paper:

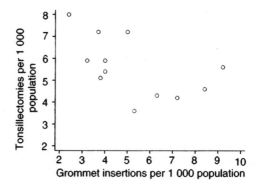

12.5.1   What does Spearman's rank correlation measure and why was it used in this situation in preference to the usual product-moment correlation coefficient?

12.5.2   What does the value -0.59 tell us about the relationship between the two rates?

12.5.3   Why would we be wrong to conclude that inserting grommets prevent tonsillectomy?

ANSWERS

12.4.3 The difference is reported as 'n.s.', meaning 'not significant'. All we know is that the probability of getting a difference as big as this if the null hypothesis were true is greater than 0.05. It could be as small as 0.06, or as big as 0.9. This makes it difficult to judge the strength of the evidence. It would be better to quote the exact probability.

12.4.4 For a two-sample t test, data in the two populations being compared should follow Normal distributions with the same variance. The SIP data do not do this. The distributions appear highly skew and the standard deviations are very different in the two groups. The Asthma School group has only 32 subjects, which is too few for a large sample approximation to be valid, especially in view of the extreme skewness.

12.4.5 We are comparing two independent groups with data which could not be transformed to a Normal distribution because most of the observations are zero. A Mann–Whitney U test would be appropriate here. It may be that the authors did not have access to the indivual SIP scores on the reference sample, but only to the aggregated means and standard deviations, which would prevent this.

12.5.1 Spearman's rank correlation, rho, measures the strength of relationship between two variables which need only be ordinal. It gives a value between -1 and $+1$, where 0 means no relationship. Spearman's rank correlation measures any association between the two variables and does not necessarily require it to be linear. It is used here because the calculation of the product-moment correlation coefficient with a 95% CI requires that both variables follow a Normal distribution. We can see that both grommet and tonsillectomy rates are skew.

12.5.2 There is a negative relationship of moderate size between grommet insertion and tonsillectomy rates.

12.5.3 This study is an ecological study where relationships are investigated at the area level. These analyses are thus not performed at the level of individuals and so any associations observed may be indirect. Hence we can only conclude that high grommet insertion rates are associated with low tonsillectomy rates within areas but cannot conclude anything about associations at the individual level.

QUESTIONS

12.6 In a study of adenoidal obstruction in children, degree of mouth breathing and speech hyponasality were rated on a four-point scale (none = 1, mild = 2, moderate = 3, marked = 4). The ratings were averaged for each child to give a nasal obstruction index. Lateral soft tissue roentgenograms were classified as showing either no obstruction, borderline obstruction, or obstruction. The results for 1 033 children considered for tonsillectomy and/or adenoidectomy are shown in the following table of frequencies:

Nasal obstruction index	Roentgenographic findings			Total
	No obstruction	Borderline obstruction	Obstruction	
1.0	454	19	55	528
1.5	124	13	33	170
2.0	65	5	39	109
2.5	26	1	38	65
3.0	19	10	63	92
3.5	3	2	25	30
4.0	0	1	38	39
Total	691	51	291	1 033

The authors reported Kendall's tau b = 0.51, $P < 0.0001$ (Paradise *et al.* 1998).

12.6.1 What is meant by Kendall's tau b? What does the 'b' signify?

12.6.2 Why is Kendall's tau b appropriate to see whether these two ratings are related? What does 0.51 indicate?

12.6.3 What would be the effect on tau b if a sample of children from the general population were used instead?

12.7 In a study of factors influencing survival in patients needing dialysis, a risk stratification system was devised, putting patients in three groups: high, medium, and low risk. This was compared to another risk classification, which also classified patients as being of high, medium, or low risk. The concordance between the two stratifications was moderate (Kendall's tau c = 0.60) (Chandna *et al.* 1999).

12.7.1 Why would Kendall's rank correlation be used here rather than Spearman's?

12.7.2 Why is the unusual tau c form used?

ANSWERS

12.6.1 Kendall's tau b is a rank correlation coefficient. It measures the extent to which ordering by each of two variables would arrange the observations into the same numerical order. Kendall's tau exists in three variants, of which tau b is the one most often used. In this form two variables may give a perfect correlation even though there are some observations with the same numerical values, i.e. ties.

12.6.2 Both variables are ordinal rather than interval scales, and if we treated them as numerical both would be very far from the Normal, the nasal obstruction score being highly skew and the roentgenogram bimodal. Thus the usual product-moment correlation coefficient would not be suitable. There are many ties in each ranking, which indicates that Kendall's rank correlation coefficient is preferable to Spearman's rho. Tau b = 0.51 is a moderate to strong rank correlation. Values of tau tend to be smaller than those of Spearman's or the product-moment correlation coefficient, which tend to be similar to one another.

12.6.3 We would expect to get many more subjects with no obstruction on roentgenogram and a score of 1.0 on the nasal obstruction score. This would strengthen the relationship between the two rankings and increase tau b.

12.7.1 Kendall's rank correlation handles ties in a better and more explicit way than does Spearman's. There are many ties here, so Kendall's would be preferred.

12.7.2 There are three forms of Kendall's tau: tau a, tau b, and tau c. The choice of which to use depends on whether a perfect relationship would give tau = 1 for the type of data being considered. Kendall's tau a = 1 only if the two rankings order each pair in the same way. The denominator for tau a is the total number of pairs. Ties in either ranking prevent perfect correlation being achieved. Kendall's tau b is adjusted for the number of ties, the denominator being reduced when ties are present. It is possible for tau b to be one, even when ties are present, provided observations tied on one ranking are tied on the other. Kendall's tau b can be used for contingency tables with ordered variables, as we have here, but can only achieve tau b = 1 when the number of rows and columns are equal, i.e. when the table is square. Kendall's tau c was specifically developed for contingency tables and can achieve tau c = 1 even when the numbers of rows and columns differ (Kendall 1970).

13
The analysis of cross-tabulations

To investigate the relationship between two qualitative variables, we tabulate one variable by the other to get a table of frequencies. This is a contingency table. We can use a chi-squared test to test the null hypothesis that in the population there is no relationship between the two variables. This compares the observed frequencies with those expected if the null hypothesis were true. This is a test for large samples; a guide to the validity for small samples is that at least 80% of the expected frequencies should exceed 5.0, all expected frequencies should exceed 1.0.

When the sample is too small, we can combine or remove rows and columns until the validity condition is met. For a 2×2 table we can use Fisher's exact test or Yates' continuity correction to the chi-squared test. There is a very computer-intensive version of Fisher's exact test for tables larger than 2×2.

We can take the ordering of categories into account using the chi-squared test for trend and related methods. When we wish to compare proportions in matched samples we use McNemar's test, a version of the sign test. We can test whether data are consistent with a theoretical distribution using the chi-squared goodness of fit test. A special case of this, the Poisson heterogeneity test, is used to test whether a set of frequencies could have the same population mean.

The odds of an event is the ratio of the probability of the event to the probability that the event does not occur. In a 2×2 table of disease (yes or no) by exposure to risk factor (yes or no) the odds ratio is the ratio of the odds of exposure if disease is present to the odds of exposure if the disease is absent. This is the same as the ratio of the odds of disease if exposed to the odds of disease if not exposed, and is given by the ratio of cross-products. In a case–control study, the risks of disease cannot be estimated, because we start with the disease not the risk factor. We cannot estimate the relative risk directly. We can calculate the odds ratio, which is a good estimate of the relative risk if the disease is rare in the population (as most diseases are).

QUESTIONS

13.1 The table below is taken from a study investigating the cause of diarrhoea in patients with gastroenteritis and shows the relationship between foreign travel and a positive result for the organism *Providencia alcalifaciens* (Haynes and Hawkey 1989):

Recent travel abroad?	P. alcalifaciens Positive (no.)	P. alcalifaciens Negative (no.)	Total
Yes	25	229	254
No	5	368	373
Total	30	597	627

$$\chi^2 = 23.98, P < 0.001.$$

13.1.1 What kind of study is this?

13.1.2 What is meant by '$\chi^2 = 23.98$, P < 0.001?'

13.1.3 Explain briefly how the chi-squared test works.

13.1.4 What conditions do the data have to meet for the test to be valid?

13.1.5 What conclusions can be drawn from these data?

13.1.6 What other information would be useful in deciding whether *P. alcalifaciens* was a likely cause of gastroenteritis in travellers?

ANSWERS

13.1.1   This is a cross-sectional study. There is a single group of patients and both assessments, *P. alcalifaciens* and travel history, were made at the same time.

13.1.2   This is the result of the chi-squared test which tests the null hypothesis that there is no association between *P. alcalifaciens* and foreign travel. The value 23.98 is the test statistic which will follow a Chi-squared distribution with 1 d.f. if the null hypothesis is true. $P < 0.001$ tells us that the probability of these data or more extreme data occurring if the null hypothesis were true is smaller than 0.001 and so we have good evidence that the null hypothesis is not true and conclude that an association exists (*Intro* §13.1).

13.1.3   The chi-squared test works by comparing the observed frequencies with those expected if the null hypothesis were true. If the null hypothesis were true then the observed and expected frequencies would be similar. Hence, a large value of the test statistic indicates good evidence against the null hypothesis. The actual value is looked up in a table of the Chi-squared distribution to give the exact probability of a value greater than or equal to that observed (*Intro* §13.1).

13.1.4   The chi-squared test is a large sample test and the usual rule is that the large sample approximation holds if all expected frequencies are greater than 5 for a 2 × 2 table. Although one observed frequency is 5, no expected values will be as small. This is because if the null hypothesis were true then the overall probability of being positive for *P. alcalifaciens* would be $28/627 = 0.04$ and this proportion would apply to those who have and those who have not travelled abroad. Thus, the expected numbers positive for *P. alcalifaciens* would be $254 \times 28/627 = 11.3$ for those who have travelled abroad and $373 \times 28/627 = 16.7$ among those who have not travelled abroad. The other expected values can be calculated in a similar way but will be large because the expected values must add to the marginal totals for each row and column (*Intro* §13.3).

13.1.5   The study shows that there is a statistically significant association between travelling abroad and being positive for *P. alcalifaciens* among people with gastroenteritis. We cannot conclude from this that *P. alcalifaciens* was the cause of the gastroenteritis. We can only conclude that an association between *P. alcalifaciens* and foreign travel exists.

13.1.6   We need a control group. We could look at the number of positive screens for *P. alcalifaciens* among subjects without diarrhoea cross-classified according to whether or not they had recently travelled abroad. This would tell us if the observed association between travel and *P. alcalifaciens* was a general one or one specific to those with diarrhoea.

QUESTIONS

13.2   In a study of the use of alternative medicines, households were randomly selected from Adelaide and country centres in south Australia. Three thousand and four people were interviewed; 48.5% of respondents used at least one non-prescribed alternative medicine. Significantly more females used alternative medicines than males (55% versus 42%, $\chi^2 = 50.0$, d.f. = 1, P < 0.001) (MacLennan *et al.* 1996).

13.2.1   What conclusions can we draw from this study about differences between Australian men and women in their use of alternative medicines?

13.2.2   What conclusions can we draw from this study about the use of alternative medicines elsewhere?

13.3   In a trial of maternity care (Turnbull *et al.* 1996), pregnant women were randomized to shared care or midwife-managed care, the following results were given:

Mode of delivery	Shared care number (%)	Midwife care number (%)	
Spontaneous	440 (73.7%)	450 (73.5%)	P = 0.9
Instrumental	86 (14.3%)	83 (13.6%)	
Emergency caesarean	55 (9.2%)	60 (9.8%)	
Elective caesarean	16 (2.7%)	19 (3.1%)	

13.3.1   What method could be used to calculate P = 0.9 and why is it appropriate?

13.3.2   What conditions do the data have to meet for the test to be valid?

13.3.3   What conclusions can we draw from this study?

13.4   In a study of patients admitted to an otolaryngology ward, 140 patients with nose-bleeds were compared to 113 controls with other conditions. Patients were interviewed about their alcohol consumption (McGarry *et al.* 1994). The results were:

Alcohol consumption	Nose-bleed patients (n=140)	Other patients (n=113)	Significance
Non-drinkers	47 (34%)	39 (35%)	
Occasional drinkers	30 (21%)	40 (35%)	
Regular drinkers	63 (45%)	34 (30%)	P < 0.025

The authors stated that 'The proportion of non-drinkers in the patients with nose bleeds was similar to that in the controls (34% versus 35%), but the proportion of regular drinkers was significantly higher (45% versus 30%, P < 0.025, χ^2 test of proportions.)' What is wrong with this statement and what analysis should they have done?

ANSWERS

13.2.1   We can conclude that in the population from which this sample was drawn, women are more likely to use alternative medicines than men. These were sampled from Adelaide and country centres in south Australia and thus the gender difference observed might not be generalizable to the whole of Australia.

13.2.2   We cannot draw any conclusions about the use of alternative medicines elsewhere from this study.

13.3.1   The data here are qualitative and are displayed as a contingency table. Therefore, the chi-squared test would be appropriate. This method tests the null hypothesis that there is no association between mode of delivery and type of care. The test gives a probability, or P value, which indicates the strength of evidence against this null hypothesis (*Intro* §13.1). A small P value indicates strong evidence.

13.3.2   For the test to be valid, 80% of the expected frequencies should be greater than 5 and all expected frequencies greater than 1. Here, there are eight frequencies altogether and so we would need to have at least seven expected frequencies to be greater than 5. This condition will be fulfilled because there are similar numbers in both modes of care and all modes of delivery have at least 16 observations (*Intro* §13.3).

13.3.3   The P value is very large, much greater than the usual cut-off of 0.05 and so we have no evidence for an association between mode of delivery and type of care. Hence we would conclude that in the population from which these subjects come, there is no evidence that providing shared care or midwife-managed care affects the distribution of mode of delivery. We can draw a conclusion about causation because this is a randomized controlled trial.

13.4   The authors appear to have tested each line of the 3×2 contingency table separately. This would involve doing three significance tests using the same data. This increases the chance of a type I error, a significant difference where there is none in the population. The authors could have done a chi-squared test for a 3×2 contingency table. This would have ignored the order of the consumption categories and so a chi-squared test for trend would be preferable which takes the ordering into account (*Intro* §13.1, 13.8).

QUESTIONS

13.5   Blood from 471 male volunteers aged 18–65 years was tested for antibodies to *Helicobacter pylori* (Webb *et al.* 1994). Seroprevalence of *H.
pylori* increased with age as shown in the following table:

	Age group						
	< 30	30–34	35–39	40–44	45–49	50–54	55–65
Seropositive	22	26	14	30	32	23	29
Seronegative	52	55	59	53	31	28	17
% Seropositive	30%	32%	19%	36%	51%	45%	63%

For trend, $\chi^2 = 20.6$, $P < 0.001$.

➕ 13.5.1   What is a trend test and how would you interpret the one presented
here?

➕ 13.5.2   What would be the advantages and disadvantages compared to a chi-
squared test for a contingency table?

➕ 13.5.3   Suggest an alternative way of testing the difference in seropositivity in
the two groups assuming that the raw data were available.

13.6   Panic disorder, panic attacks and other psychiatric disorders were
assessed in a random sample drawn from five US communities (Weissman *et al.* 1989). The following table shows odds ratios for previous
suicide attempts for the three categories of psychiatric patients compared to non-psychiatric controls.

	Panic disorder	Panic attacks	Any other psychiatric disorder	No psychiatric disorder
Odd ratio	24.9	13.5	6.3	1.0
95% CI	17.5 to 35.5	10.1 to 18.1	5.1 to 7.8	

13.6.1   What is meant by an odds and an odds ratio?

13.6.2   What would you conclude from the odds ratios given here?

❗ 13.6.3   Why is the odds ratio for no psychiatric disorder equal to 1.0 and why
has it no confidence interval?

ANSWERS

13.5.1 The trend test is the chi-squared test for trend. It works by assigning numerical values to each category and then estimating the regression of one variable on the other. Here, that would essentially mean that we plot the proportions seropositive by age and test for a straight line fit. The chi-squared test for trend tests the null hypothesis that the slope of this line is zero. The calculated χ^2 value is 20.6 on 1 d.f. with an associated P value smaller than 0.001. This provides strong evidence for a trend in the proportions and so we would conclude that the proportion of males who are seropositive increases with age (*Intro* §13.8).

13.5.2 The test for trend takes into account the ordering of the age groups, which the ordinary contingency table chi-squared does not. Hence, the test for trend has much greater power to detect a steady increase (or decrease) in seropositivity with age. However, the test has less power to detect non-linear relationships, such as seropositivity being higher among young men and older men than among those in the middle of the age range. Such a relationship would produce a non-significant trend test.

13.5.3 Assuming that age was recorded in years and given the large samples (176 seropositive, 295 seronegative), we could compare the difference in mean age between the two groups using the large sample comparison (z test) (*Intro* §9.7).

13.6.1 The odds of an event is the ratio of the probability of the event to the probability of the event not happening, that is $p/(1 - p)$ if p is the probability of the event. The odds ratio gives the odds in one group relative to another group and is a measure of the magnitude of association between the variables, here psychiatric category and previous suicide. In a 2×2 table of frequencies, the odds ratio is given by the ratio of the cross-products (*Intro* §13.7).

13.6.2 Here, the odds ratios compare each psychiatric group with the control group. All odds ratios are greater than one showing that the odds of a previous suicide are greater in every psychiatric category than in the control group. The highest odds ratio is for panic disorder and the lowest for disorders not associated with panic. We conclude that in the population from which the sample was drawn, there is a positive association between previous suicide attempts and a diagnosis of psychiatric disorder. We can also conclude that the odds for suicide are greater for panic disorder and panic attacks than for other psychiatric disorders combined as the confidence intervals do not overlap.

13.6.3 The psychiatric groups are all compared to this group and so its odds ratio is one by definition. It is not an estimate and so has no confidence interval.

QUESTIONS

13.7   Forty-five alcoholic patients and 23 non-alcoholic research or laboratory
staff were studied. A two allele polymorphism was identified and subjects were classified into three genotypes, AA, AB and BB (Sherman
et al. 1993). The following table was produced:

Genotype	Alcoholic subjects	Non-alcoholic subjects
BB	19	2
AB	19	3
AA	7	18

$$\chi^2 = 25.8, \text{ d.f.} = 2, \text{ P} < 0.001.$$

13.7.1   What does '$\chi^2 = 25.8$, d.f. $= 2$, P < 0.001' tell us about the relationship
between alcoholism and genotype?

13.7.2   What additional analysis would be useful?

13.8   In a study of diet and epithelial ovarian cancer, 235 women with cancer and 239 women from the general population were interviewed about
consumption of milk products; 49% of cancer patients and 36% of controls reported consuming yoghurt at least monthly, relative risk $= 1.7$,
P $= 0.01$. Questions were asked about six other milk products, none
of which gave a significant difference, nor was there an overall tendency
for cancer patients to consume more of these products (Cramer *et al.*
1989).

13.8.1   What is meant by relative risk and what technique could be used to
calculate it in this study?

13.8.2   How would the findings about other milk products influence the conclusions drawn from the study?

13.9   Infants who died from sudden infant death syndrome (SIDS) or cot
death were compared to a group of live infants, matched for age and
birthweight. Infants who died were more likely than live infants to have
been laid to sleep in the prone position (odds ratio 4.58, 95% CI 1.48 to
14.11) (Ponsonby *et al.* 1992).

How would you interpret the odds ratio of 4.58 and the confidence interval in this study?

ANSWERS

13.7.1   This is the result of a chi-squared test on the 2×3 table. It tests the null hypothesis that there is no association between alcoholism and genotype. The alternative hypothesis is the general one of an (unspecified) association. Since $P < 0.001$, there is strong evidence against the null hypothesis and we conclude that there is an association. However, the nature of the association is not given by the test (*Intro* §13.1).

13.7.2   It would be helpful to quantify the association. This could be done by calculating odds ratios for say AB versus AA and BB versus AA. These together with 95% CIs would provide estimates of the nature of the relationship with a measure of precision. The table below shows the odds ratios for being alcoholic:

Genotype	Odds ratio (95% CI)
BB	24.4 (4.5 to 133.5)
AB	16.3 (3.6 to 72.9)
AA	1.0

This shows that the alcoholics are more likely to be AB than AA and are even more likely to be BB (*Intro* §13.7).

13.8.1   Relative risk is the ratio of the risk of having the disease among those with the factor (yoghurt eating) to the risk of having the disease among those negative for the factor (non-yoghurt eaters). This is a case–control study and so the relative risk cannot be calculated directly but is estimated by the odds ratio (or cross-product ratio). This will give a good estimate of the true relative risk because the disease, epithelial ovarian cancer, is rare (*Intro* §8.6).

13.8.2   It affects the interpretation of the difference. If this is one of several significance tests it may be the 1 in 20 which would be significant by chance and thus may be spurious. If we apply a Bonferroni correction we would multiply the P values by 7, because there are 7 tests and the difference would not be significant. The findings also suggest that there is no risk from milk products in general (*Intro* §9.10).

13.9   This is a case–control study where the condition of interest, cot death, is a rare event. Hence, the odds ratio will be a good estimate of the relative risk of death for babies laid to sleep in the prone position compared to other positions. We conclude that in the population from which this sample was drawn, babies laid to sleep in the prone position are more likely to die of cot death than babies laid to sleep on their backs. The wide confidence interval suggests that this risk could be as great as 14-fold but might only represent a 50% increase in risk (*Intro* §13.7). We should not conclude that changing the baby's position will reduce the risk of cot death. We could get these results if there were some other factor related to both choice of sleeping and infant death.

QUESTIONS

13.10 Sixty-three suicide cases and 63 matched controls were compared to investigate factors related to suicide among discharged psychiatric patients. Matching was by age, sex, clinical diagnosis and date of admission. Data on cases and controls was extracted from hospital notes (Dennehy *et al.* 1996). The table below shows some of the results:

Clinical and social variables	No. of suicide cases	No. of controls	P value	Odds ratio (95% CI)
Duration of illness < 5 years	35	24	0.09	1.9 (0.9 to 4.2)
Relapsing illness	19	14	0.34	1.6 (0.6 to 4.0)
Past dangerous self harm	27	19	0.20	1.7 (0.8 to 4.0)
Past self-harm	44	38	0.34	1.6 (0.70 to 3.7)
Depressed at last contact	22	13	0.11	1.9 (0.8 to 4.8)
Communicated ideas of suicide	33	15	0.004	4.0 (1.6 to 12.0)
Alcohol or drug misuse	26	27	1.00	1.0 (0.3 to 3.3)
Unemployed	47	49	0.83	0.9 (0.4 to 2.3)
Married	12	19	0.14	0.4 (0.1 to 1.3)

➕ 13.10.1 What statistical test could be used to derive the P values in the table? What null hypothesis is being tested?

❗ 13.10.2 The authors reported that 'many clinical and social variables thought to be associated with suicide did not distinguish cases and controls'. What information in the table has led to this conclusion?

13.10.3 Comment on any drawbacks of the study design.

ANSWERS

13.10.1 The data are one-to-one matched with a yes/no outcome. Hence we have proportions in two matched samples and should use McNemar's test. This tests the null hypothesis that the proportion of suicides with the factor is the same as the proportion of controls with the factor. Matching on diagnosis may be important, as both suicide and the possible risk factors may be related to it. We should not ignore it (*Intro* §13.9).

13.10.2 The P values have led to this conclusion. Of the 10 clinical and social factors examined, only one shows a statistically significant result, communicating ideas of suicide. This factor is associated with a four-fold increase in odds of suicide. Although no other factors are significant, several show odds ratios in the 'expected' direction, for example short duration of illness and past depression are associated with a nearly two-fold increase in odds. Also the confidence intervals indicate that the population odds ratios could be quite large. Not significant does not mean that no association exists (*Intro* §9.6).

13.10.3 Associations were observed but were mostly non-significant because of the small sample size. The study was retrospective with data being taken from hospital notes. It is possible that the information taken from the hospital notes was of poor quality which might have weakened the associations observed. For example, it may be that communication of ideas of suicide was not always recorded. In addition, the suicide cases were matched to the controls for age, sex, clinical diagnosis and date of admission. This matching may have reduced some of the differences between cases and controls such as for duration of illness and relapsing illness, where these factors may be related to the diagnosis. It would have been interesting to investigate differences in diagnoses but since the study matched cases and controls according to this variable, this cannot be investigated.

QUESTIONS

13.11   Bland *et al.* (1979) carried out a questionnaire study of cigarette smoking and respiratory symptoms among secondary school children. The sample was all children in the first year of a random sample of secondary schools in Derbyshire. Children were asked questions about their respiratory symptoms and their parents were also asked about the child's symptoms. The following data were presented:

Cough first thing in the morning

Reported by the child's parents	Reported by the child			Total
	Yes	No	Not known	
Yes	29	104	0	133
No	172	5 097	8	5277
Not known	6	132	0	138
Total	207	5 333	8	5548

Two tests of significance were given: a chi-squared test for association ($\chi^2 = 119.4$, d.f. $= 1$, $P < 0.001$) and McNemar's test ($\chi^2 = 16.3$, d.f. $= 1$, $P < 0.001$). Both tests were done using continuity corrections. The 'not known' row and column represented cases where the question was not answered. They were omitted from the tests.

⊕ 13.11.1   Why are two different values of chi-squared given? What is each testing?

⊕ 13.11.2   Do you think it was correct to omit cases where either answer was unknown?

⊕ 13.11.3   Was the use of continuity corrections necessary?

⊕ 13.11.4   What can we conclude?

❶⊕ 13.11.5   What aspect of the data did the statistician ignore in these analyses, which compromises the validity of these tests?

ANSWERS

13.11.1 The first test, for association, is the usual contingency table chi-squared test. It tests the null hypothesis that there is no relationship between symptoms reported by parents and children. The second test, McNemar's test, tests the null hypothesis that there is no difference in the proportion of parents reporting the symptom and the proportion of children reporting the symptom, (*Intro* §13.1, 13.9).

13.11.2 We do not know why the question was not answered. It may be that the respondents were not sure what was meant by terms such as 'usually' and 'first thing in the morning' and so felt unable to reply. As the authors were not interested in whether lack of understanding or knowledge by parents and children were related, they decided to omit subjects with incomplete data. An alternative approach, used in other parts of the study, would be to take the variable as being that a cough was reported or not reported, and combine the 'not known' and 'no' categories. The analysis described here gives the same answer either way.

13.11.3 Although the numbers are quite large, the expected frequency in the 'yes, yes' cell is small: $133 \times 201/5402 = 4.9$ ('not knowns' omitted from totals). Thus a continuity correction is required by the conventional criterion of at least 80% of expected frequencies must exceed five, which means all of them in a 2×2 table. For the McNemar's test the relevant expected frequencies are in the 'yes, no' and 'no, yes' cells, which are both large (128.1 and 196.1), so a continuity correction is not essential. However, it is arguable that continuity corrections should always be used in preference to uncorrected chi-squared tests as they make the Chi-squared distribution fit the exact distribution better, and by the same argument the exact distribution is always better than the chi-squared, corrected or not (*Intro* §13.5, 13.9).

13.11.4 There is evidence that the child's report and the parent's report are related, i.e. if the child reports the symptom, the parent is more likely to report the symptom than if the child does not report the symptom. However, this relationship is not close, and most positive reports by children are not corroborated by their parents. Children are more likely to give a positive report than are their parents.

13.11.5 Martin Bland ignored the clustering. Children were sampled by school, and members of a school may be more like one another than they are like members of another school. Hence the observations are not truly independent, as they should be for both these tests. There are several ways in which the clustering could be taken into account, e.g. by logistic regression using school as a categorical predictor variable (*Intro* §2.11, 11.12, 17.8).

QUESTIONS

13.12 In a retrospective study of ovarian irradiation in breast cancer, the case records of 29 patients treated with a radiation dose of 12 Gy were compared with 31 patients treated with 14 Gy. Of these, patients above 40 years of age had fewer ovarian ablation failures with the 14 Gy schedule than with 12 Gy ($0/12 = 0\%$ and $2/14 = 14\%$, respectively) although the difference was not statistically significant ($P = 0.56$, Fisher's exact test) (Leung *et al.* 1991). The authors reported that the overall ablation failure rate in younger patients was unacceptably high at 35% (12/34) compared to 8% (2/26) in older patients ($P = 0.02$, chi-squared test).

13.12.1 What is meant by Fisher's exact test and why was it used here?

13.12.2 What can we conclude from the result?

13.12.3 Comment on the design of the study as a comparison of dosage regimes and as a comparison of age groups.

13.13 In an analysis of all deaths associated with volatile substance abuse in UK, the number of deaths associated with the abuse of aerosols over a 10-year period were reported as follows:

Year	Deaths	Year	Deaths
1988	46	1993	11
1989	24	1994	2
1990	31	1995	5
1991	27	1996	11
1992	11	1997	8

The authors reported a Poisson heterogeneity test, giving $\chi^2 = 98.89$, d.f. $= 9$, $P < 0.00001$. The expected frequencies were found from the total number of deaths divided by the total number of years, $176/10 = 17.6$ (Taylor *et al.* 1999).

✚ 13.13.1 What null hypothesis is being tested?

✚ 13.13.2 What can we conclude about deaths associated with aerosol abuse?

✚ 13.13.3 What aspect of the calendar is ignored here? How could this be corrected?

ANSWERS

13.12.1 Fisher's exact test is a method of testing the null hypothesis that for patients above 40 years of age the proportion of failures on the two regimes is the same, in the population from which these patients come. It works as follows. Each possible table which could give the observed row and column totals is constructed and the probability of it arising under the null hypothesis is calculated. The sum of the probabilities for the observed table and all tables with frequencies further from those expected under the null hypothesis are added to give $P = 0.56$. Fisher's exact test can be used for any 2×2 table, but is particularly useful when the expected frequencies are small. Here two of the four expected values are less than 5 and so the chi-squared test cannot be used (*Intro* §13.4).

13.12.2 We have failed to show that there is a difference in failure rate, but cannot say that there is no difference (*Intro* §9.6).

13.12.3 This is an observational study. Women were not randomly allocated to dosage, which we would usually expect for the comparison of two treatments. Thus, there may be differences between the women which have led to their being given different treatments, and which may in turn lead to differences in outcome which are not due to treatment. It may also be that a change in treatment followed a change in personnel, and there may be other features of treatment which have also changed. Thus, we should be reluctant to draw any definitive conclusions from such a comparison. The sample size is quite small, and far too small to be expected to detect any differences between two rather similar treatments when the outcome variable is dichotomous. This is shown by the observed difference, 0% versus 14%, which is not significant (although it is quite large). For the comparison of age groups, we cannot randomize. Observational studies are all that is possible.

13.13.1 The null hypothesis is that the annual rate at which deaths occur is constant (*Intro* §13.10).

13.13.2 We can conclude that the annual rate of deaths is not constant. The number of deaths has declined greatly over the 10-year period. This coincided with a change in propellant from chloro-fluoro-carbon (CFC) compounds to butane, as CFCs were phased out to reduce damage to the ozone layer (*Intro* §13.10).

13.13.3 The years 1988, 1992, and 1996 were leap years and so had one extra day on which deaths could take place. The total number of days was thus, $7 \times 365 + 3 \times 366 = 3\,653$. We could allow for this by making the expected numbers of deaths $176 \times 366/3\,653 = 17.63$ for the leap years and $176 \times 365/3\,653 = 17.59$ for the other years. The adjustment would make very little difference (*Intro* §13.10). This approach also ignores any changes in the population at risk over this period.

14
Choosing the statistical method

Many statistical problems involve one of the following:

- the comparison of two means of a continuous variable,

- the relationship between two quantitative variables,

- the relationship between two qualitative variables.

Most data can be described as being one of the following types of scale:
- ratio, where the ratio of two quantities has a meaning, e.g human height,

- interval, where the difference between observations has a meaning, though their ratio may not, e.g. calendar year,

- ordinal, where we can order subjects from lowest to highest, e.g. anxiety score,

- ordered nominal, where subjects are grouped into several categories, which have an order, e.g. tumour stage,

- nominal, subjects are grouped into categories which need not be ordered in any way, e.g. eye colour,

- dichotomous, subjects are grouped into only two categories, e.g. survived or died.

The types of comparison and variable guide us as to which statistical method to use. For example, to compare two groups with an ordinal variable we could use the Mann–Whitney U test. To compare matched groups on a ratio scale we could consider the paired t method.

QUESTIONS

14.1   Lung function and prevalence of respiratory symptoms were compared between 42 cross-country skiers and 29 non-skiing controls (Larsson *et al.* 1993). Forced expiratory volume in 1 s (FEV1) was recorded as the percentage of that expected given age, sex and height. Abnormal shortness of breath and other symptoms were recorded at an interview. Some results are shown in the table:

	Number of subjects	FEV1 (% expected)		Abnormal breathlessness	
		Mean	SD	Yes	No
Skiers	42	112	11	17	25
Non-skiers	29	105	14	4	25
		P<0.05		P<0.02	

14.1.1   What method should be used to test the null hypotheses that skiers and non-skiers have the same mean FEV1? What conditions do the data have to fulfil for the test to be valid?

14.1.2   What method should be used to test the null hypotheses that skiers and non-skiers have the same prevalence of abnormal breathlessness? What conditions do the data have to fulfil for the test to be valid?

14.1.3   What conclusions can be drawn about skiing, lung function and respiratory symptoms?

14.2   In a double-blind comparison of two ointments, containing calcipotriol or betamethasone, for the treatment of psoriasis, 345 subjects were given one ointment on the left side of the body and the other on the right, the side being chosen at random. The severity of the condition was assessed by self report as 'cleared', 'pronounced improvement', 'slight improvement', 'no change', or 'worse', and by visual assessment as a score by the investigator.

The score was significantly lower (P < 0.001) for the calcipotriol side than the betamethasone side. Patients were more likely to report 'cleared' or 'pronounced improvement' on the calcipotriol side (Kragballe *et al.* 1991).

14.2.1   Suggest three methods which could be used to carry out the significance test on the scores. What assumptions would be required for each?

14.2.2   The self-assessment was recoded into two categories, 'cleared or pronounced improvement' or 'little or no improvement'. What methods could be used to carry out the significance test for the recoded data?

14.2.3   What can we conclude?

14.2.4   What method could be used without collapsing the five categories into two, as in 14.2.2 above?

ANSWERS

14.1.1 We could use the two-sample t test. We are comparing two independent small samples and the variable is on an interval scale. The data should come from populations which follow Normal distributions with the same variance. These conditions will be satisfied since FEV1 is approximately Normal, and the standard deviations are not very different (*Intro* §14.3).

14.1.2 This can be done by a chi-squared test for a 2×2 table, or by a Normal comparison of two proportions. We are comparing two independent samples and the variable is dichotomous. For either method, all expected frequencies must be greater than 5. Since the samples are quite small, we could use Yates' correction to the chi-squared test or use Fisher's exact test (*Intro* §14.3).

14.1.3 We can conclude that cross-country skiers tend to have better lung function and are more likely to have abnormal breathlessness than non-skiers. (The theory is that this is the result of breathing very cold air during exertion.)

14.2.1 The data are paired. The score may or may not be an interval level measurement. If it is interval then the paired t test could be used. This would require that the differences come from a Normal distribution. We could also do a large sample z test, which would not require this assumption. The results would be the same. The Wilcoxon paired test could also be used but this would be less powerful than the t test if the t test assumptions were satisfied. The assumption would be that the score is an interval level variable. If we did not wish to treat the score as interval, we could use the sign test which simply requires us to specify what direction a difference is in, hence requires only ordinal data (*Intro* §14.4).

14.2.2 The data are paired and the variable is dichotomous. We could use McNemar's test to compare the proportions who had improved for the two treatments (*Intro* §14.4).

14.2.3 The response was better using calcipotriol ointment than using betamethasone, though we are not told by how much. As this was a randomized double-blind trial, the evidence suggests that the ointment itself was the cause.

14.2.4 We could use the sign test. For each subject we can say whether the category is better, equal or worse on the calcipotriol side than on the betamethasone side (*Intro* §14.4).

QUESTIONS

14.3   In a study of birth position in labour, 218 women were randomly allocated to squatting using a birth cushion and 209 to conventional management. Fourteen percent of women did not use the position to which they had been allocated. The squatting group had significantly fewer forceps deliveries and significantly shorter mean duration of labour (Gardosi *et al.* 1989).

14.3.1   Suggest a method which could be used to test the statistical significance of the difference in forceps deliveries.

14.3.2   Suggest a method which could be used to test the statistical significance of the difference in the mean duration of labour.

14.4   In a study of prevalence of headache and migraine in schoolchildren, a 10% random sample of the children in each school in a city was taken. The estimated prevalence of migraine was 10.8% (95% CI 9.1 to 12.3%). Children with migraine and one age- and sex-matched control for each were invited for interview and clinical examination. The mean number of days lost from school was 7.8 (range 0–82) among 159 children with migraine and 3.7 (range 0–42) among their matched controls. Asthma was present in 18.2% of migraine sufferers and 12.6% of their controls (Abu-Arefeh and Russell 1994).

14.4.1   What statistical techniques might be considered for the investigation of the difference in lost school days, and what considerations would influence the choice of an appropriate method?

14.4.2   What statistical technique could be used to investigate the difference in asthma?

14.5   In a study of prostitution and the risk of HIV, one hundred and ninety three female prostitutes were examined for acute sexually transmitted disease and of these 27 had one or more current infections (Ward *et al.* 1993). The following table shows the proportion of prostitutes with acute sexually transmitted infection by the number of non-paying sexual partners:

No. of non-paying partners	Proportion (%) with acute sexually transmitted infection
0	3/38 (8%)
1	17/107 (16%)
> 1	7/25 (28%)

What statistical test could be used to investigate the relationship between number of sexual partners and prevalence of sexually transmitted infections?

ANSWERS

14.3.1   We have proportions from two independent samples. If the number of forceps deliveries is large enough, we can use the chi-squared test or the large sample comparison of proportions. These two methods will give the same P value. We could also use Fisher's exact test which is valid for any 2×2 table (*Intro* §14.3).

14.3.2   We have two independent samples and a ratio scale of measurement. We are not given any information about the distribution of duration of labour, however, the two groups in this study are large and so the means will follow a Normal distribution. Hence we can use the large sample Normal test to compare mean duration of labour in the two groups (*Intro* §14.3).

14.4.1   We have a paired comparison and a ratio scale. The variable must have a highly skew distribution because the mean is much closer to the minimum than maximum value. We can also see from the ranges that the variability increases with the mean. The sample is quite large, and matched. We could consider a paired t test or a paired large sample z test, using the case and matched control as the pair. Although the sample is quite large, the highly skew distribution will lower the power of this test. We could try to transform to a Normal distribution, but we cannot use a simple logarithm because of the zeros. A square root may be appropriate. It is likely that no transformation will work because of the discrete nature of the variable and large number of zeros that might be present. A rank test, the Wilcoxon matched-pairs signed-rank test could be used. This would be suitable because the variable is an interval scale of measurement. The sign test could also be used, but would be less powerful in a sample as large as this. The disadvantage of these methods is that they will not give confidence intervals without making very strong assumptions about the data (*Intro* §14.4).

14.4.2   We have a paired comparison with a dichotomous variable. McNemar's test would allow for the matching. A matched odds ratio could also be used. A chi-squared test for a contingency table or a comparison of two independent proportions by the large sample Normal test would ignore the matching, which might be important as age and sex are important in childhood asthma (*Intro* §14.4).

14.5   The data are qualitative and the number of partners is ordered. Hence, we should use the chi-squared test for trend. This gives $\chi^2 = 4.4$, d.f. $= 1$, P $= 0.035$, which is statistically significant, thus providing evidence for a trend in prevalence with the number of non-paying sexual partners (*Intro* §14.5).

QUESTIONS

14.6   Life expectancy at birth for nine developed countries was plotted against percentage of national income received by the least well-off families (Wilkinson 1992):

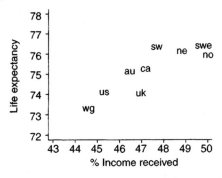

Key: wg=West Germany, us=United States, au=Australia, uk=United Kingdom, ca=Canada, sw=Switzerland, ne=Netherlands, swe=Sweden, no=Norway.

What method of analysis could be used to estimate the strength of relationship between life expectancy and income?

14.7   In a study of a possible diagnostic test for urothelial malignancies, responses obtained from cellular extracts from 8 patients with urothelial cancer and 28 controls with normal bladders were compared (Stoeber *et al.* 1999). A figure similar to this was presented:

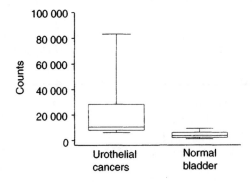

14.7.1   What does the graph tell us about the shapes of the distributions?

14.7.2   The groups were compared using an 'equal variance t test'. Do you think this approach is acceptable here?

14.7.3   What possible approaches could be used to compare these groups?

ANSWERS

14.6   We are investigating the relationship between two continuous, interval scale variables. We could use regression, correlation, or rank correlation (*Intro* §14.5). The data look like a reasonable fit to the Normal distribution, so rank correlation would not be indicated here. The author used a correlation coefficient to estimate how strongly the two variables were related in the population from which the samples were drawn. The actual correlation is 0.86, $P < 0.001$ which shows that there is a strong positive association between life expectancy and equality of income distribution at the level of the country. This does not show, of course, that equalizing income would help people live longer. This is an ecological study and the results are at the level of the country (*Intro* §3.10).

14.7.1 The shapes of the distributions appear to be positively skew. The upper half of the box is bigger than the lower half and the upper whisker is much longer than the lower whisker.

14.7.2 There appears to be a huge difference in variability between the two groups. The assumption that they are samples from populations with the same variance does not seem plausible.

14.7.3 The groups are small and we have interval data. We could try a transformation, such as the log, and then use the two-sample t method. We could also use the Mann–Whitney U test (*Intro* §14.3). After the problem with their analysis had been pointed out, the authors used the latter approach. This, not surprisingly, was highly significant, $P = 0.0002$ (Hales and colleagues, unpublished personal communication to *Lancet*).

15
Clinical measurement

In this chapter we consider a number of topics related to issues of measurement in medicine.

Almost all measurements are made with some error. We can measure this in two ways: using the within-subject standard deviation and other statistics derived from this, such as the repeatability, and using the intraclass correlation. The first helps us to interpret the individual observation, the second tells about the general properties of the measurement method. We can compare two different methods of measuring the same thing by the 95% limits of agreement, based on differences between measurements made on the same subject using the two methods.

We can investigate how good a diagnostic technique is using the sensitivity, the proportion of cases of the disease correctly identified, and the specificity, the proportion of cases without the disease correctly identified. A plot relating sensitivity to specificity is called a receiver operating characteristic (ROC) curve and the probability that someone positive on the test actually has the disease is called the positive predictive value. The positive predictive value depends on the prevalence of the disease.

The limits within which observations from most normal people will lie, the reference interval or normal range, can be estimated from mean ± two standard deviations, provided the distribution is a close approximation to the Normal. If not, the distribution can often be transformed to be suitable.

Survival data can present special problems in analysis because some subjects, still surviving, have unknown survival times. Life table techniques and the Kaplan–Meier survival curve can be used to describe survival and survival in different groups can be compared using the log-rank test.

The number needed to treat is a way of describing the results of a clinical trial. It is the number of patients we would have to treat with the new treatment to save one extra life or achieve one more successful outcome compared to the effects of the old treatment. Although intuitively attractive, we must be careful interpreting it when the difference is not significant or the new treatment is less successful than the old.

QUESTIONS

15.1   In Africa, serological testing for HIV infection is both expensive and
difficult to obtain and so a study sought to assess the value of regional
lymph node enlargement, by site and by size, as a predictor of HIV
disease (Malin *et al.* 1994). The sensitivities and specificities were given
as follows:

Site (size (cm)) of lymph node	Sensitivity (rate (%))	Specificity (rate (%))	Odds ratio 95% CI
Axillary (≥1)	63/146 (43)	107/113 (95)	13.5 (5.3 to 36.6)
Axillary (≥0.5)	110/146 (75)	78/113 (69)	6.8 (3.8 to 12.3)
Submandibular (≥1)	31/146 (21)	109/113 (96)	7.4 (2.4 to 25.4)
Submandibular (≥0.5)	110/146 (75)	84/113 (74)	8.9 (4.9 to 16.3)
Epitrochlear (≥1)	53/146 (36)	102/113 (90)	5.3 (2.5 to 11.5)
Epitrochlear (≥0.5)	123/146 (84)	92/113 (81)	23.4 (11.7 to 47.6)
Epitrochlear (≥0.5) +axillary (≥1)	63/146 (43)	108/113 (96)	16.4 (6.0 to 48.6)
Epitrochlear (≥0.5) +submandibular (≥1)	31/146 (21)	111/113 (98)	15.2 (6.1 to 42.0)
Axillary (≥1) +submandibular (≥1)	34/146 (23)	111/113 (98)	16.9 (3.8 to 104.0)
Epitrochlear (≥0.5) +axillary (≥1) +submandibular (≥1)	26/146 (18)	112/113 (99)	24.3 (3.4 to 488.5)

15.1.1   What are the sensitivity and specificity of a test? What do they tell us?

➕ 15.1.2   How could we present the sensitivity and specificity graphically?

➕ 15.1.3   What does the odds ratio tell us here?

The positive and negative predictive values were also given:

Site (size (cm)) of lymph node	Positive predictive value (rate (%))	Negative predictive value (rate (%))
Axillary (≥1)	63/69 (91)	107/190 (56)
Axillary (≥0.5)	110/145 (76)	78/114 (68)
Submandibular (≥1)	31/35 (89)	109/224 (49)
Submandibular (≥0.5)	110/139 (79)	84/120 (70)
Epitrochlear (≥1)	53/64 (83)	102/195 (52)
Epitrochlear (≥0.5)	123/144 (85)	92/115 (80)
Epitrochlear (≥0.5) +axillary (≥1)	63/68 (93)	108/191 (57)
Epitrochlear (≥0.5) +submandibular (≥1)	31/33 (94)	111/226 (49)
Axillary (≥1) +submandibular (≥1)	34/36 (94)	111/223 (50)
Epitrochlear (≥0.5) +axillary (≥1) +submandibular (≥1)	26/27 (96)	112/242 (46)

15.1.4   What are positive and negative predictive values and on what do they
depend?

ANSWERS

15.1.1   The sensitivity is the proportion of subjects with disease whom the test
         detects. It tells us how good the test is at finding the disease. The
         specificity is the proportion of subjects without disease whom the test
         correctly identifies. It tells us how good the test is at excluding people
         who do not have the disease (*Intro* §15.4).

15.1.2   We could draw the ROC curve. This is a plot of the sensitivity versus
         1 − specificity for each possible cut-off, with the points joined up (*Intro*
         §15.4).

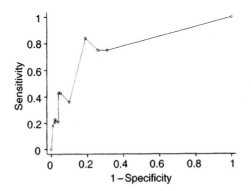

15.1.3   It tells us the strength of the relationship between the diagnostic test
         and HIV disease. As all the CI are well away from 1.0, there is good
         evidence that all tests are related to HIV (*Intro3* §15.4).

15.1.4   The positive predictive value is the proportion of those subjects who
         are identified as diseased by the diagnostic test, who actually have the
         disease. It depends on the prevalence of the disease, increasing as preva-
         lence increases. The negative predictive value is the proportion of those
         subjects who are identified as not having the disease (i.e. as being HIV
         negative) by the diagnostic test who actually do not have the disease
         (i.e. really are HIV negative). It also depends on the prevalence of the
         disease, decreasing as prevalence increases (*Intro* §15.4).

QUESTIONS

15.1.5   Why are the denominators constant in the sensitivity and specificity columns but varying in the positive predictive value column?

15.1.6   Why does the sensitivity go up and the specificity go down if we reduce the size of node which we consider positive?

15.1.7   Which two diagnostic tests give the strongest relationship to HIV and how do they differ?

15.2   Stell and Gransden (1998) investigated two tests for sepsis in bursitis, comparing 17 patients with septic bursitis to 19 patients with non-septic bursitis. One test was the culture of aspirated fluid in liquid media. The test was positive in all 17 cases of septic bursitis and negative in 17 of the 19 cases of non-septic bursitis. They quoted the specificity, the proportion of non-septic bursitis cases correctly identified, as 89% (95% CI 74 to 104%) and the sensitivity, the proportion of septic bursitis cases correctly identified, as 100% (95% CI 92 to 108%).

15.2.1   How do we know that these confidence intervals are wrong?

15.2.2   What should they have done?

15.3   In a discussion of testing for HIV the child of an HIV positive mother, the following appeared: 'These tests are not "notorious for false positives". It is well known that they may produce them, but the reliability increases in high prevalence situations.' (Talbot 1999).

In what sense does the reliability of a test increase as the prevalence increases and how is this relevant to testing such a child?

ANSWERS

15.1.5   The denominator for sensitivity is the number HIV positive, the denominator for specificity is the number HIV negative. These are the same for all the tests. The denominator for positive predictive value is the number positive on the test, which varies from test to test. Similarly, the denominator for negative predictive value is the number negative on the test, which also varies from test to test (*Intro* §15.4).

15.1.6   Lowering the cut-off point makes more subjects test positive, while still including all those test positive at the higher cut-off. This increases the numerator of the sensitivity, while the denominator is constant, thus automatically increasing the sensitivity. It therefore also reduces the number test negative and reduces the specificity (*Intro* §15.4).

15.1.7   The biggest odds ratios are for the combination of epitrochlear ≥ 0.5 cm and axillary ≥ 1 cm and submandibular ≥ 1 cm, odds ratio = 24.3, and for epitrochlear ≥ 0.5 cm, odds ratio = 23.4. The combined test has low sensitivity, only 18%, though it has a high specificity (99%). It does not find many cases, but those found are very likely to be HIV positive (positive predictive value = 96%). The epitrochlear ≥ 0.5 cm test has higher sensitivity, 84%, and also a fairly high specificity (81%). It would find most of the cases, and those found are fairly likely to be HIV positive (positive predictive value = 85%). It is thus, the preferred test (*Intro* §15.4).

15.2.1   Specificity and sensitivity cannot exceed 100%, so the confidence intervals cannot exceed 100% either (*Intro* §15.4).

15.2.2   Because the numbers are so small, they should use an exact confidence interval based on the binomial probabilities. This requires a computer program (e.g. StatExact, or our free program Biconf, from www.sghms.ac.uk/depts/phs/staff/jmb) or chart (Pearson and Hartley, 1970, p. 228). The 95% CI is for sensitivity 0.80 to 1.00 (80 to 100%) and for specificity 0.67 to 0.99 (67 to 99%). Note that for specificity the confidence interval cannot include 100%, because we have observed a test positive in the sample of true negatives (i.e. non-septic bursitis cases) and so we know that not all tests are negative and 100% is impossible (*Intro* §8.4, 8.8).

15.3   As the prevalence of the disease increases the positive predictive value increases and the negative predictive value decreases. Thus a positive test is more likely to indicate the presence of the disease when the prevalence is high. As this child is a member of a high-risk population, a positive test would make the probability of HIV infection being present very high indeed (*Intro* §15.4).

QUESTIONS

15.4   The normal, reference or 95% range for haematocrit in men is 0.39–0.55 (Lentner 1984).

15.4.1   What is meant by this statement?

15.4.2   What would it tell us about a man with a haematocrit of 0.47?

15.4.3   What would it tell us about a man with a haematocrit of 0.38?

15.4.4   What would it tell us about a woman with a haematocrit of 0.38?

15.4.5   If the range was calculated from the mean and standard deviation of haematocrit measured in 100 men, what assumptions were made? What other method could be used, and what would be its advantages and disadvantages?

15.5   In a study of 52 kidney transplant patients, 24 had primary non-function (i.e. the transplanted kidney did not function immediately). The paper reported plasma calcium, phosphate and immunoassayable parathyroid hormone (i-PTH) concentration before transplantation in patients with primary function and non-function (Varghese *et al.* 1988). The results were presented as follows:

	Plasma calcium (mmol/L) mean (SE)	Plasma phosphate (mmol/L) mean (SE)	i-PTH (ng/L) (normal range < 1 200) mean (SE)
Primary function	2.50 (0.04)	1.64 (0.09)	1 760 (330)
Primary non-function	2.56 (0.04)	1.78 (0.10)	3 069 (389)
P value *	NS	NS	< 0.01

* Unpaired t test.

15.5.1   What is meant by the term 'normal range < 1 200'?

15.5.2   What would you conclude about i-PTH in kidney transplant patients?

ANSWERS

15.4.1 A reference range is a range of values within which 95% of observations will lie assuming that the individuals included are 'normal', i.e. without any specific pathology. Thus, in this example, we can say that 95% of men will have a value of haematocrit between 0.39 and 0.55. Thus, 5% of 'normal' men will have values which lie outside the range (*Intro* §15.5).

15.4.2 A man with haematocrit 0.47 is 'normal' as far as haematocrit is concerned, although he may be 'abnormal' in other ways (*Intro* §15.5).

15.4.3 A man with haematocrit 0.38 has a value which is outside the reference range and so is rather low, although it is not far below the lower limit. This might indicate some 'abnormality' or he could just be one of the 5% outside (*Intro* §15.5).

15.4.4 From the reference range given we can conclude nothing about a woman with haematocrit 0.38 since the reference range is for men only. In fact the reference range given for women is 0.36–0.48 (Lentner 1984), so this is within the reference range for women (*Intro* §15.5).

15.4.5 The assumptions would be that haematocrit follows a Normal distribution and that the mean and standard deviation are reasonably well estimated. The symmetrical 95% limits would then be mean-1.96SD to mean$+1.96$SD. The other method is to estimate the range from the frequency distribution directly, taking the 2.5 and 97.5 percentiles. The advantage is that no assumption of Normality is required but the disadvantage is that it is less accurate when the Normal distribution assumption is correct (*Intro* §15.5).

15.5.1 The normal range for i-PTH is a range of values which would include 95% of supposedly healthy individuals and is calculated by taking two standard deviations either side of the mean, assuming a Normal distribution. Here, only the upper limit is given and suggests that a value over 1 200 would be regarded as unlikely in a healthy person (*Intro* §15.5).

15.5.2 The mean value for both groups of transplant patients was over 1 200, showing that these patients tend to have higher levels than healthy patients. The significance test shows that there is good evidence for a difference in mean levels between those with primary function and those with primary non-function. The standard deviations can be calculated from the SE to be $330 \times \sqrt{28} = 1\,746$ and $389 \times \sqrt{24} = 1\,906$. The distributions are, therefore, positively skew, but it is unlikely that there are no observations at all below 1 200, particularly in the primary function group. This suggests that some kidney transplant patients may have apparently 'normal' levels of i-PTH, particularly those with subsequent primary function (*Intro* §15.5).

QUESTIONS

15.6   In Mid Downs Health Authority a register of babies born with cystic
fibrosis was kept from 1962 to 1991. During that time 32 babies were
born of whom seven have died. The following Kaplan–Meier survival
curve shows their survival (Tom Scanlon, personal communication)

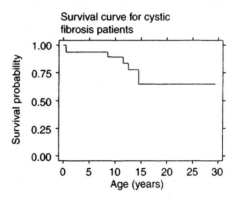

15.6.1   Why is the Kaplan–Meier survival curve appropriate?

15.6.2   What does this graph tell us about the survival of cystic fibrosis babies?

15.7   A study investigated the prognostic value of P53 antibodies in 353 uns-
elected primary breast cancer patients. P53 antibodies were detected in
42 cases (12%). The median duration of follow up for live patients was
5.3 years. Overall survival in the group with and without P53 antibodies was compared using a log-rank test. Survival was worse in patients
with P53 antibodies ($P < 0.0005$) (Peyrat *et al.* 1995).

15.7.1   What is the log-rank test for and what feature of the data makes the
authors use this technique?

15.7.2   What question does the test try to answer and what conclusion would
you draw?

15.8   A review article on the treatment of acute ischaemic stroke contained a
statement that thrombolysis reduced the risk of being dead or dependent
at the end of the studies reviewed. The absolute risk reduction (ARR)
was 4.2%, (95% CI 1.2 to 7.2%) and the number needed to treat (NNT)
was 24 (95% CI 14 to 83) (Gubitz and Sandercock 2000).

15.8.1   What is meant by 'absolute risk reduction'?

15.8.2   What is meant by 'number needed to treat'?

15.8.3   What is the relationship between NNT and ARR?

ANSWERS

15.6.1   The babies are born at different times during the 30-year period and are therefore followed up for different lengths of time. In addition, some babies died. This method allows us to use the data from each subject from their birth to the end of the study or their death if this occurred during the follow-up period, making allowance for the different lengths of follow up.

15.6.2   We can see that between 1962 and 1991 in Mid Downs Health Authority, the majority of babies survived for at least 10 years and the 30-year survival rate was about 60% (*Intro* §15.6).

15.7.1   The log-rank test is a method of comparing survival in two groups of patients. It allows for the possibility that some subjects have not yet died and that subjects have been followed for varying lengths of time (*Intro* §15.6).

15.7.2   The test tries to determine the evidence for a difference in survival between patients with and without P53 antibodies in breast cancer patients as a whole. The P value is very small and so we have strong evidence that patients without P53 antibodies survive longer than patients with P53 antibodies in the population from which the sample was taken (*Intro* §15.6).

15.8.1   The ARR is the difference in the proportion of patients dying or dependent without thrombolysis and the proportion of patients dying or dependent after receiving thrombolysis. It is the difference between two proportions. It is given here as a percentage.

15.8.2   The NNT is the number of patients we would have to treat with thrombolysis to prevent one patient dying or being dependent (*Intro3* §15.9).

15.8.3   To show this relationship, we need to represent ARR as a difference between two proportions rather than between two percentages, i.e. ARR = 0.042. Then NNT = 1/ARR, i.e. 1/0.042 = 23.8. This is usually given as an integer, 24 (*Intro3* §15.9).

QUESTIONS

15.9   A study was carried out to determine whether computer assisted analysis of lung area on the chest radiograph reliably predicted lung volume in neonates. Chest radiographs taken for clinical purposes were scanned and analysed using imaging software and the lung area was calculated. This was compared with lung volume, assessed by measurement of functional residual capacity (FRC) using a helium gas dilution technique, within 1 hour of the chest radiograph being performed. Fifty infants, median gestational age 30 weeks (range 24–43), were studied (Dimitriou et al. 1999).

To determine the repeatability of the lung area measurements, the first 20 radiographs were assessed independently by two observers and by the first observer on two separate occasions. The mean lung area calculated by the first observer was 11.8 cm^2 (SD = 4.8) and of the second was 11.7 cm^2 (SD = 4.9). The mean difference between observers was 0.07 cm^2 (range −0.83 to 1.15). The interobserver coefficient of repeatability was 1.06 cm^2. The difference between the measurements of lung area made by two observers was plotted against the mean of the two observers' measurements (two data points are overlapping):

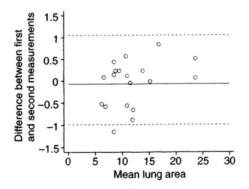

The first observer re-evaluated the radiographs; the mean lung area calculated on the second occasion was 11.69 cm^2 (SD = 4.66). The mean difference between the two calculations was 0.1 cm^2 (range −1.07 to 0.94). The intraobserver coefficient of repeatability was 1.0 cm^2.

15.9.1   What is the coefficient of repeatability? How can the intraobserver coefficient of repeatability of 1.0 cm^2 be interpreted?

15.9.2   What is the purpose of the figure?

15.9.3   What can we deduce about the effect of using a different observer to measure lung area?

ANSWERS

15.9.1 The coefficient of repeatability is calculated either from twice (or 1.96 times) the standard deviation of the differences or from $2\sqrt{2}$ (or $1.96\sqrt{2}$) times the within subject standard deviation. We expect that 95% of differences between pairs of measurements will be less than the repeatability. Thus, we expect that if pairs of measurements are made on the same infant by the same observer, 95% of such pairs of lung areas will be closer than $1.0\,\mathrm{cm}^2$ (*Intro* §15.2).

15.9.2 The figure is to investigate whether the measurement error between the observers can be assumed to be uniform, or varies with the magnitude of the measurement. Here, the number of observations is small, but there is nothing to suggest that the observations become more widespread as the lung area increases (*Intro* §15.2).

15.9.3 The intraobserver repeatability coefficient was $1.0\,\mathrm{cm}^2$, the interobserver repeatability coefficient was $1.06\,\mathrm{cm}^2$. Thus, the differences when two different observers measured were more variable by only a tiny amount. The observer makes very little difference to the precision.

QUESTIONS

The median lung area of the 50 infants was $11.23\,cm^2$ (range 0.82–28.53) and their median FRC was 28 ml (3–103). Lung area correlated significantly with lung volume (Spearman's correlation coefficient = 0.60, $P < 0.001$). No other analysis or graph was given.

⊕ 15.9.4   Why did the authors use the Spearman rank correlation coefficient?

❶⊕ 15.9.5   What other analysis might be preferable?

❶⊕ 15.9.6   The authors' conclusion was that 'computer assisted analysis of the chest radiograph lung area is a reliable method of assessing lung volume in neonates.' Is this supported by the results?

15.10   In a study of the measurement of muscle strength, tests were carried out on 20 healthy subjects, 5 men and 15 women aged between 60 and 84, by two observers. Among others, isometric tests were carried out on elbow and knee. The results were presented in two ways: as ICC and as within-subject standard deviations, for which the authors used the term 'standard error of measurement (SEM)'. Each was calculated for observations by the same observer, intra-rater, and for observations by two different observers, inter-rater (Richardson *et al.* 1998).

⊕ 15.10.1   What do ICC and SEM each tell us about the measurement error?

The following results were given (measurements in kgf):

	Intra-rater			Inter-rater		
	ICC	(95% CI)	SEM	ICC	(95% CI)	SEM
Elbow	0.88	(0.75, 1)	1.57	0.87	(0.78, 1)	1.67
Knee	0.89	(0.76, 1)	1.84	0.67	(0.44, 1)	3.16

❶⊕ 15.10.2   What can we conclude about the measurement of muscle strength using this dynamometer?

ANSWERS

15.9.4   Both measured lung area and lung volume have positively skew distributions, as shown by the median being nearer to the lower end of the range than to the upper. Thus neither variable follows a Normal distribution. For a correlation coefficient we need Normal data. They could either use a transformation, such as the logarithm, or use a method which is unaffected by skewness. They chose the Spearman rank correlation coefficient (*Intro* §12.4).

15.9.5   A plot of lung volume against lung area would help to show how closely the two measurements were related. Regression of lung volume against area, using a logarithmic transformation, would enable us to predict volume from area, with a 95% CI for the predicted lung volume (*Intro* §11.6).

15.9.6   It would be reasonable to conclude that the measurement of lung area is repeatable. Two measurements of lung area are unlikely to be more than $1\,cm^2$ apart, which is small compared to the standard deviation of measured area, almost $5\,cm^2$. However, the authors only present a rank correlation between measured volume and lung area. The correlation is highly significant and there is strong evidence that a relationship exists in the population. The correlation is not very high, however, and evidence of a relationship is not the same as evidence of a reliable prediction. This correlation does not indicate a close relationship. Correlation is not usually very helpful in comparing different methods of measurement (*Intro* §15.3).

15.10.1 ICC tells us about the information content of the measurement. The closer to 1.00 the ICC is, the more information it contains. The SEM tells us about the interpretation of an individual measurement on a subject. It tells us 95% of measurements will be within $1.96 \times$ SEM of the subject's average value, and that 95% of pairs of measurements on the same subject will differ by less than $1.96 \times \sqrt{2}$SEM (*Intro* §15.2).

15.10.2 For the elbow measurement, we can conclude from the ICC that the elbow measurement has quite a high degree of repeatability and that it does not matter which observer makes the measurement. From the SEM, the observed value is likely to be within 3 ($= 1.96 \times 1.57$) kgf of the subject's average value. For the knee measurement, the repeatability is quite high provided the same observer is used, but it is not so good if different observers make the measurements. For a given observer, the measurement is likely to be within 3.6 ($= 1.96 \times 1.84$) kgf of the average measurement on that subject by the same observer, but only within 6.2 ($= 1.96 \times 3.16$) kgf if either observer might be used (*Intro* §15.2).

QUESTIONS

!⊕ 15.10.3 The upper 95% confidence limits for ICC are all given as 1. Why must this be wrong?

⊕ 15.10.4 The authors comment that the results suggest that the two raters' techniques were different for the knee but not for the elbow. Do you agree?

Muscle strength varied considerably in the sample:

	Range	Mean	SD
Elbow	1.8–18.8	7.8	4.9
Knee	9.2–35.4	19.11	6.3

!⊕ 15.10.5 The authors commented that the variation between subjects contributed to the size of the reliability coefficient. Why is this? Does it affect the SEM?

⊕ 15.10.6 What shape does the distribution of muscle strength have? Does this affect the results in any way?

!⊕ 15.10.7 What would be the best way to improve the study?

ANSWERS

15.10.3 If the population ICC = 1, then each observation on a subject will be the same. We know that this is not true in the sample, so it cannot be true in the population from which the sample comes. Hence the upper 95% confidence limit must be less than 1 (*Intro* §15.2).

15.10.4 For the elbow, there is virtually no difference in the ICC or the SEM for the intra-rater and inter-rater error. Using different raters does not add any variability. For the knee, there is a big difference. Using a different rater produces a substantial extra error. It is reasonable to conclude that they are not measuring the same thing, and since the patient has not changed to conclude that the observers are not measuring in the same way (*Intro* §15.2).

15.10.5 The ICC is calculated from the variance between subjects divided by the sum of the variances between and within subjects. The variance within subjects is fixed and the variance between subjects depends on the sample. Thus a very variable sample will produce a big ICC. The ICC is only meaningful for the population for which our subjects form a representative sample. The variability between-subjects does not affect the SEM because this relies on the within-subject standard deviation (*Intro* §15.2).

15.10.6 Both must be positively skew (skew to the right). There are two clues to this. First, the mean is closer to the lower end of the range than to the upper end. Second, the standard deviation is too large for symmetry. For the elbow it is greater than half the mean, implying negative values, and for the knee the mean minus twice the standard deviation is considerably less than the lower limit of the range. Correlation coefficients are difficult to interpret when the variables do not follow a Normal distribution, because we cannot easily calculate a valid confidence interval. There is therefore some doubt over the ICCs.

15.10.7 We are drawing conclusions about whether observers can agree from a sample of only two observers. The study would be improved by increasing the number of observers. We could also add more subjects, but it is the observers who are critical (*Intro* §15.2).

16
Mortality statistics

The risk of dying depends very strongly on age and sex, so the comparison of mortality between different populations must take their age and sex distributions into account. Mortality is usually analysed separately for males and females. Mortality rates can be presented as crude rates which ignore the age distribution, or as a series of age-specific rates for narrow age groups.

When the population is large and there are many deaths in every age group, the mortality rates can be compared using the direct method of age standardization. In this we use a standard age structure and work out what mortality rate this standard population would have if the age-specific mortality rates of each of the populations to be compared applied to it.

When there are few deaths, we use age standardization by the indirect method. In this we have a standard set of age-specific mortality rates. We calculate the number of deaths we would expect in the populations to be compared if they experienced these standard age-specific mortality rates. We divide the actual number of deaths observed by the expected number to give the standardized mortality ratio. This is often multiplied by 100.

Yet another way of comparing mortality is the demographic life table. This is calculated from age-specific mortality rates applied to an imaginary group of people followed from birth to death. The expectation of life is the average number of years members of this imaginary group would live. Expectation of life can be calculated at any age. Expectation of life at birth depends greatly on mortality rates in the early years of life. It should not be thought of as the age at which most people die, a common misunderstanding.

QUESTIONS

16.1 The graph below shows life expectancy at birth for nine developed countries plotted against percentage of national income received by the least well-off families (Wilkinson 1992).

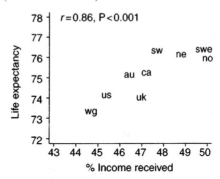

Key: wg=West Germany, us=United States, au=Australia, uk=United Kingdom, ca=Canada, sw=Switzerland, ne=Netherlands, swe=Sweden, no=Norway.

16.1.1 What is meant by 'life expectancy at birth'? What data are used in its calculation?

16.1.2 To what aspect of mortality is life expectancy particularly sensitive?

16.1.3 Can we conclude that unequal distribution of income causes reduction in life expectancy?

16.2 'They say life begins at 40. Not so long ago, that's about when it ended.' This was the heading of an advertisement produced by the Association of the British Pharmaceutical Industry. The advertisement claimed that, had we lived in the 19th century, we would have attended many funerals of people who died aged about 40. This was because expectation of life was 40 years for men and 42 years for women (St. George 1986).

16.2.1 Were they right?

The advertisement went on to point out that in the late 20th century this did not happen, expectation of life having increased greatly. The conclusion was that this increase in life expectancy was because of advances in pharmaceuticals as a result of animal experimentation.

16.2.2 Was this a reasonable conclusion?

ANSWERS

16.1.1   Life expectancy at birth is a way of summarizing a set of age-specific death rates. It is the average number of years which would be lived from birth, if these age-specific mortality rates were to apply throughout life. It is calculated from a life table, which shows what would happen to a hypothetical birth cohort if these age-specific mortality rates applied. Life expectancy can be used for comparing mortality between populations or over time (*Intro* §16.4).

16.1.2   Because it is the average number of years lived since birth, it is particularly sensitive to mortality in the early years of life. Two populations with different life expectancy may only differ in infant mortality rates (*Intro* §16.4).

16.1.3   No, this is an observational, ecological study. We have showed only that in countries where the percentage of income received by the least well-off families is lower, that life expectancy tends to be lower (*Intro* §16.4).

16.2.1   Expectation of life is the average number of years people would live under the current age-specific mortality rates, not the number of years that most people will live. In the 19th century death rates were highest at very young ages, particularly the first year, and in the later years from 60 onwards. Most people died as young children or in old age, so the average life span was about 40 years, but this was not the peak age at death. Males who reached 15 years had an average remaining life of 43 years, longer than the average life span at birth. In the 20th century death rates in childhood fell greatly, so that by 1999 male life expectancy at birth was 74 years, increased by 34 years since 1841, and at age 15 it was 59 years, increased by only 14 years since 1841. Most of the extra years of life were due to children surviving into adulthood (*Intro* §16.4). N.B. St. George (1986) criticized the advertisements, he did not originate them!

16.2.2   It is true that gains in life expectancy came over the same period that modern pharmaceuticals were developed, but this does not mean that one caused the other. Many other changes took place over the same period, such as improvements in midwifery, sanitation, housing, nutrition, and education. All of these may have had a part to play. Many other less likely things changed, too. Bombs became bigger and more destructive, for example, but we might be reluctant to conclude that the gains in life expectancy were due to that.

QUESTIONS

16.3   Researchers developed a new method of expressing survival in cancer patients using the fraction of remaining life span. In reply to a letter about their paper they wrote that 'when we say that a woman aged 40 has a life expectancy of 75 we mean that the cumulative probability of her dying by age 75 is 100%, not 50% (median survival) as Tan assumes.' (Vaidya and Mittra 1997, 1998, Tan 1997)

Do you agree with the authors explanation of 'life expectancy'?

16.4   In a study of post-natal suicide among mothers in England and Wales, the standardized mortality ratio (SMR) for suicide among women who had just had a baby was 17 with a 95% CI 14 to 21 (women aged 15–44 years, England and Wales, 1973–87, SMR for all women = 100). For women who had had a still birth, the SMR was 105 (95% CI 31 to 277) (Appleby 1991).

16.4.1   What is meant by 'standardized mortality ratio'?

16.4.2   Why are SMRs used in the study of mortality?

16.4.3   How would you interpret the 95% CI 31 to 277?

16.4.4   What conclusions can be drawn from the study?

ANSWERS

16.3   Life expectancy is the average number of years to be lived. This is
        calculated from summing all the years of life from a given time point
        for a group of people and dividing by the number of people. If the life
        expectancy for a woman aged 40 were 75 then this would mean that on
        average women lived a further 75 years beyond 40. Assuming that the
        authors meant that the life expectancy was 75 years from birth, then
        even this does not mean that all women die by age 75, it means that 75
        is the average length of life. Some women will by definition live shorter
        and some longer than this (*Intro* §16.4).

16.4.1 A SMR is the result of the indirect method of standardizing mortality
        for age. This method is used when the number of deaths is too small
        to estimate age-specific mortality rates reliably. If we know the age
        structure of the observed population we can indirectly compare this
        death rate with that of a standard population as follows. The number
        in each age group in the observed population is multiplied by the age-
        specific mortality rates from a standard population to give the numbers
        of expected deaths. Adding these gives the total number of expected
        deaths for the observed population. We divide the number of observed
        deaths by the expected deaths and multiply by 100 to get the SMR
        (*Intro* §16.3).

16.4.2 We use SMRs because the risk of dying from most conditions depends
        on age. Populations which differ in age distribution will therefore differ
        in mortality, even if the risks for any given age are the same. Here
        the proportion of women aged over 40 in the new mother population
        would be much less than in the general population, for example. By
        standardizing we obtain an estimate of the difference as it would be
        if the age distributions were the same. The SMR method is good for
        small populations and rare causes of death, because we do not have to
        estimate age-specific mortality rates (*Intro* §16.3).

16.4.3 The 95% CI is from 31 to 277. This means that the data are consistent
        with an SMR as small as 31 or as large as 277 among women experiencing
        still birth (*Intro* §8.3).

16.4.4 We can conclude that women who had just had a baby were less likely
        than women in general to commit suicide, the risk being between 14%
        and 21% of that for all women of the same age. Women who had had a
        still birth had a greater risk than other mothers, because the confidence
        intervals do not overlap. However, they could have a greater or smaller
        risk than women in general, since the confidence interval includes 100.

QUESTIONS

16.5   The following table contains data from an investigation of leukaemia registration and death in people under 25 years of age in UK local authority
areas with at least one-third of the population within 10 miles of one
of 14 nuclear installations and control areas by grouping of installation.
Registration and mortality rates were both standardized using the indirect method (Gardner 1989).

Outcome	Standardized ratios		Installation to control area ratio (95% CI)
	Installation area	Control area	
Leukaemia registration	112	97	1.15 (1.03 to 1.30)
Leukaemia mortality	102	107	0.95 (0.85 to 1.08)

❗ 16.5.1   What is meant by the standardized ratio of 112 for registration for all
installation areas and the standardized ratio of 97 for the corresponding
control areas?

❗ 16.5.2   The ratio of these standardized registration ratios is 1.15 with 95% CI
1.03 to 1.30. What additional information does the confidence interval provide about the comparison between the installation and control
areas?

❗ 16.5.3   What would you conclude about the evidence for an excess risk of
leukaemia in installation areas?

16.6   In a study of melanoma in Australia, a representative sample of 30 976
adult subjects were asked whether they had ever been treated by a doctor for skin cancer. The diagnosis was then obtained from the treating
doctor or hospital (Giles *et al.* 1988). The authors calculated an incidence rate per 100 000 people per year, standardized for age and sex to
the world population.

16.6.1   What does this mean and what information was required to do it?

16.6.2   Is this the direct or indirect method?

ANSWERS

16.5.1   The standardized ratio 112 tells us that the rate of a leukaemia regis-
         tration was 12% higher in installation areas than in the UK population
         in general. In control areas, the rate of leukaemia registration was 3%
         less than for the UK in general. Hence it appears that registration was
         more common in installation areas (*Intro* §16.3).

16.5.2   The ratio directly compares the two standardized ratios and the 95% CI
         tells us about the precision of this comparison. The data are consistent
         with a true ratio of standardized ratios as small as 1.03 or as big as 1.30.
         Since this interval excludes 1.0, the ratio is significant at the 5% level
         and provides evidence for a real difference in registration rates between
         installation and control areas (*Intro* §8.3).

16.5.3   There is evidence for a difference in leukaemia registration between
         installation and control areas but not for death where the ratio of stan-
         dardized mortality ratios is less than one and the confidence interval
         includes 1.0. These results might be due to greater tendency to register
         leukaemia rather than an increase in incidence in installation areas than
         in control areas.

16.6.1   The incidence of melanoma varies according to age and sex and different
         populations have different age/sex structures. Standardization enables
         us to compare rates in different countries, while taking this variation into
         account. The method of standardization uses a standard age and sex
         structure and applies the age–sex-specific incidence rates in the observed
         population. The incidence rate is multiplied by the proportion in each
         age/sex group. The sum of these is the age and sex standardized inci-
         dence rate, and provides a summary rate which can be compared with
         other similarly standardized rates (*Intro* §16.2).

16.6.2   This is direct standardization because the authors used the age/sex-
         specific incidence rates in their sample and so were able to compare
         these directly with the age/sex distribution for the world population. If
         they only had the total number of cases and the age/sex distribution in
         the sample rather than the age/sex-specific rates, then they would have
         had to use indirect standardization (*Intro* §16.2).

17
Multifactorial methods

The questions in this chapter cover material which would usually be found only in advanced courses.

Multiple regression is a method of investigating the relationship of a continuous variable with two or more other variables. A regression equation is calculated which predicts the mean value of the outcome variable for subjects with any given values of the predictor variables. We can test for interaction, where the effects of one predictor variable on the outcome variable depend on the level of another. We can fit non-linear relationships using polynomial regression, including several powers of a predictor variable in the equation. We can include qualitative predictor variables, such as tumour stage or social class, by using dummy variables, one for each level of the predictor variable except for a base category, to which the others are compared.

Multiple regression makes the same assumptions about the data as does simple regression. The differences between the observed value of the outcome variable and the value predicted by the regression equation should follow a Normal distribution and that the variance of these deviations should be constant throughout.

Multi-way analysis of variance is a different way of presenting multiple regression, used when all the predictors are qualitative. Analysis of covariance is another name for multiple regression when there is a mixture of qualitative and quantitative predictors.

Logistic regression is a multifactorial technique used when the outcome measure is dichotomous. The coefficients are usually presented as odds ratios. Cox regression is used when the outcome variable is survival time. The coefficients are usually presented as hazard ratios.

All regression methods can be done using stepwise methods, which automatically find the group of predictor variables which predict the outcome. The results can be difficult to interpret.

There is often more than one study of a question. Meta-analysis is a technique for combining data from all studies to give a common estimate of the treatment effect or risk. We must check that there is no heterogeneity, i.e. that we can assume that the studies are really estimating the same thing.

QUESTIONS

17.1 In a study of physical fitness and cardiovascular risk factors in children, blood pressure and recovery index (post exercise recovery rate, an indicator of fitness) were measured (Hofman and Walter 1989). Multiple regression was used to look at the relationship between systolic blood pressure and recovery index, adjusted for age, race, area of residence and ponderal index (wt/ht^2). For the boys, the adjusted regression coefficient of systolic blood pressure on recovery index was given as follows: $b = -0.086$, $SEb = 0.039$, 95% CI $= -0.162$ to -0.010.

17.1.1 What is meant by 'multiple regression analysis'?

17.1.2 What is meant by the terms 'b', 'SEb' and '95% CI'?

17.1.3 What assumptions about the variables are required for these analyses to be valid? How could these assumptions be checked? What could be done if they were not met?

17.1.4 Why was the regression adjusted?

17.1.5 What would be the effect of adjusting for race if systolic blood pressure were related to race and recovery index were not?

17.1.6 What would be the effects of adjusting for ponderal index if blood pressure and recovery index were both related to ponderal index?

ANSWERS

17.1.1 This is a statistical method used where we have a continuous outcome variable, here systolic blood pressure, and several possible predictors, here recovery index, age, race, area of residence, and ponderal index. The method estimates the relationship between the outcome and each predictor adjusting for all other predictors in the model. Here, the outcome or dependent variable is systolic blood pressure. The predictor, independent, or explanatory variables are recovery index, age, race, area of residence, and ponderal index (*Intro* §17.1).

17.1.2 'b' is the coefficient of recovery index in a multiple regression equation. It means that for two groups of subjects whose recovery index differs by one unit, and who all have the same age, race, area and ponderal index, the difference in mean systolic blood pressure will be b units. It is found by the method of least squares (*Intro* §17.1). 'SEb' is the standard error of the estimate of b. Different samples of the same size would give different estimates of b. SEb is the estimated standard deviation of the possible estimates of b. '95% CI' is the 95% CI for b. For 95% of possible samples, this range of values will include the value of b for the whole population (*Intro* §17.2).

17.1.3 The assumptions are that the differences between the observed systolic blood pressure and the systolic blood pressure predicted by the regression equation (residuals or deviations from the regression) follow a Normal distribution and that the variance of this distribution is uniform, i.e. unrelated to recovery index, age, race, area and ponderal index. The relationships should be linear. These assumptions could be checked graphically, by histogram and Normal plot of deviations, and by scatter plots of deviations against the outcome and predictor variables. Goodness of fit tests can be used. Lack of Normal distribution and uniform variance can be tackled by transformation, usually logarithmic. The testing of assumptions should be repeated on the new model (*Intro* §17.5).

17.1.4 Regression may be adjusted because the variable of interest, systolic blood pressure, is related to the adjusting variables, age, race, area, and ponderal index (*Intro* §17.1).

17.1.5 If recovery index is independent of adjusting variables, the adjustment will reduce the variability of the deviations and so make the estimate of b better, in that the confidence interval will be narrower, but the estimate will not be changed (*Intro* §17.1).

17.1.6 If recovery index is related to the adjusting variables, the adjustment will reduce or remove the spurious relationship between recovery index and systolic blood pressure produced by both being independently related to something else (*Intro* §17.1). Both the coefficient and its SE are likely to change.

QUESTIONS

17.2   In a cross-sectional study, pulmonary function and presence of respiratory symptoms of 4 320 Munich schoolchildren (aged 9–11 years) were measured, with height, weight, number of cigarettes smoked in the home daily, and the use of gas or coal for cooking or heating. Density of car traffic in the child's school district was obtained by a traffic census. The logarithm of peak expiratory flow rate (PEFR) was used in the analysis. Multiple regression analysis of PEFR showed a significant decrease of 0.71% (95% CI 1.08 to 0.33%) per increase of 25 000 cars daily (Wjst *et al.* 1993).

17.2.1   Why might the logarithm of PEFR have been used in the analysis?

17.2.2   Why was the coefficient presented in terms of a percentage decrease in PEFR?

17.3   An ecological study examined the effect of water fluoridation on tooth decay in 5-year-old children using data collected at the level of the electoral ward. The electoral wards included were in three areas where the water supply was either unfluoridated, artificially fluoridated or naturally fluoridated. A multiple linear regression model was fitted with mean tooth decay in the ward as the outcome and with predictors Jarman underprivileged area score for each ward and fluoridation status (unfluoridated, artificially fluoridated or naturally fluoridated). A high Jarman score indicates an area with high deprivation. The authors reported that there was a significant interaction between the effects of Jarman score and water fluoridation on tooth decay. A graph similar to this was given (Jones *et al.* 1997):

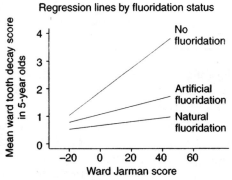

17.3.1   What is meant by interaction and how would you interpret a statistically significant interaction here?

17.3.2   This study was described as a 'natural experiment' where non-fluoridated areas acted as the control group. What problems might arise as a result of this study design?

ANSWERS

17.2.1 Logarithmic transformation is used when the distribution of the outcome variable is positively skew or when its standard deviation increases proportionally to the mean. Peak flow rate usually follows a Normal distribution for given age and sex. It may be skew here because boys and girls aged 9–11 are included, which would give quite a wide range of size of child. Also, the standard deviation of PEFR tends to increase with the mean and so will increase with age. Taking logarithms is likely to stabilize the variance and thus meet the requirement for regression analysis. Taking logs may also linearize the relationship between traffic density and PEFR (*Intro* §17.5).

17.2.2 If unlogged PEFR had been used, the regression coefficient for traffic density would indicate the change in PEFR (L/min) per unit change in traffic density. Since PEFR was logged, the regression coefficient represents the change in log(PEFR). A difference on the log scale is equivalent to a ratio on the natural scale and so the coefficient on the log scale has been antilogged to give the percentage change in PEFR per unit of traffic density.

17.3.1 An interaction between Jarman score and fluoridation status means that the relationship between mean tooth decay and Jarman score is different in areas with different levels of fluoridation. This can be seen from the graph where the regression lines for unfluoridated, artificially fluoridated and naturally fluoridated areas are not parallel. Thus, fluoridation appears to be more effective in areas of high deprivation (*Intro* §17.3).

17.3.2 Areas were not randomized to fluoridation and non-fluoridation but selected. Therefore areas not necessarily comparable. Other factors which are related to tooth decay such as lifestyle might differ between the areas. Hence, it is difficult to be conclusive about the relationship between fluoridation and tooth decay from these data.

QUESTIONS

17.4 A cross-sectional questionnaire survey was undertaken to measure the quality of care at general practice consultations. A random sample of practices was taken in four different regions of the UK and data was collected for 2 weeks on all consultations in each practice. Patient questionnaires were filled out prior to and following each consultation, and a doctor questionnaire recorded details of the consultation. The main outcome variable, enablement score, estimated the doctor's ability to 'enable' their patients and was based on patient responses to questions about the consultation. A low score indicated poor satisfaction with the consultation and a high score indicated high satisfaction. The study included 25 994 adult consultations from a total of 221 doctors in 53 practices (Howie *et al.* 1999).

The authors reported that using multiple regression at the consultation level, several covariates were identified as significant predictors of enablement. These included the patient knowing the doctor very well and the duration of consultation ($R^2 = 0.037$).

➕ 17.4.1 What is meant by 'several covariates were identified as significant predictors of enablement'

➕ 17.4.2 What further information does '$R^2 = 0.037$' provide?

➊➕ 17.4.3 The analysis was performed 'at the consultation level'. What would be the unit of analysis here? What are the advantages and disadvantages of analysing at this level rather than at the doctor or practice level?

ANSWERS

17.4.1   A covariate is a predictor variable which is related to the outcome, here enablement. Multiple regression allows us to estimate the effects of each covariate on enablement adjusting for the effects of all other covariates in the model. If a covariate is a significant predictor then we have good evidence that the association with enablement after adjusting for other covariates is real. The associated P value is probably less than 0.05.

17.4.2 R is the multiple correlation coefficient and R^2 indicates the proportion of the variance in enablement explained by the covariates in the model. Hence, only 0.037 or 3.7% of the total variation is explained in this model. This suggests that the predictive power of the covariates is low and that most of the variability remains unexplained (*Intro* §17.2).

17.4.3   The unit of analysis is one patient consultation and so in the multiple regression there is one case for each consultation i.e. 25 994 observations. Other levels are doctors ($n = 221$) and practices ($n = 53$). Here we have consultations within doctors within practices. The advantages of using consultations are that the effective sample size is larger giving a more powerful and probably a more straightforward analysis. The disadvantages are that consultations may not be independent and if this is not taken into account in the analysis we may get spurious significant results. It is hard to believe that the doctor has no effect and analysing at the consultation level is likely to lead to some difficulty in interpreting findings with respect to individual doctors.

QUESTIONS

17.5   A study in Northern Ireland compared prescribing patterns in general practices before and after the introduction of fundholding in 1993. Fundholding was a scheme whereby GPs controlled budgets with which they purchased services for their patients. The practices were analysed in four groups as non-fundholders, first, second and third wave fundholders. The table below shows the mean number of prescription items per 1 000 patients for fundholders and non-fundholders in seven successive financial years (Rafferty *et al.* 1997):

Year	Non-fund-holders (n = 268)	Fundholders		
		First wave (n = 23)	Second wave (n = 34)	Third wave (n = 9)
89–90	9 832	8 550 **	9 061 *	8 407 *
90–1	9 989	8 635 ***	9 183 *	8 567 *
91–2	10 494	8 944 ***	9 712 *	9 024 *
92–3	10 791	9 113 ***	10 143	9 342 *
93–4	11 473	9 334 ***	10 792	9 998 *
94–5	11 992	9 756 ***	11 093 *	10 423 *
95–6	12 455	10 135 ***	11 482 *	10 675 *

* $P < 0.05$, ** $P < 0.01$, *** $P < 0.001$, compared with non-fundholders.

17.5.1   The authors tested the waves and years separately. What method could be used to examine the overall effect of the fundholding group allowing for the effect of year?

17.5.2   What advantage would this approach have over individual comparisons?

17.6   A news item in the *BMJ* (Wise 1998) reported the results of a *JAMA* (Barnes and Bero 1998) study which investigated possible bias in the publication of studies of effects of passive smoking. The *BMJ* item reported that 'a review written by authors with affiliations to the tobacco industry is 88 times more likely to conclude that passive smoking is not harmful than if the review was written by authors with no connection to the tobacco industry.' This information was taken from the *JAMA* article where the following information was presented: 'In multiple logistic regression analyses ... the only factor associated with concluding that passive smoking is not harmful was whether an author was affiliated with the tobacco industry (odds ratio, 88.4; 95% CI, 16.4 to 476; $P < 0.001$)'.

17.6.1   What is meant by 'multiple logistic regression'?

17.6.2   What is wrong with the interpretation of the odds ratio by the *BMJ* writer?

ANSWERS

17.5.1 We could use two-way analysis of variance. The two variables would be fundholding status (in four groups) and year (seven groups) (*Intro* §17.7). Alternatively, we could use multiple regression with sets of dummy variables for years and waves, which would give identical results (*Intro* §17.6).

17.5.2 This would be more powerful than performing many individual comparisons because all the data would be used to estimate the random error. In addition, it would avoid the problem of over-testing the data with multiple comparisons (*Intro* §17.7).

17.6.1 Multiple logistic regression or logistic regression is a multifactorial statistical method used when we have a dichotomous outcome, here reporting passive smoking as harmful or not. The method allows us to estimate the relationship between this outcome and several predictor variables, here affiliation with the tobacco industry and others. It allows us to estimate the odds ratios for each predictor adjusted for all others in the model (*Intro* §17.8).

17.6.2 '88 times more likely' suggests that the odds ratio has been interpreted as the increase in risk, whereas it actually represents the increase in odds. These are only similar if the condition of interest is rare (see 17.6.4). Also, the odds are 87 times greater or 88 times as great rather than 88 times more likely. This is not very important here, but would be if the odds ratio were closer to 1.0 (*Intro* §13.7).

QUESTIONS

From the *JAMA* paper we can deduce the following 2×2 table for passive smoking effects by tobacco industry connections.

		Passive smoking		Total
		No effect	Harmful	
Tobacco industry	Yes	29	2	31
affiliation	No	10	65	75
Total		39	67	106

➕ 17.6.3   Just for a change, we will do some sums on this table! What is the odds ratio for concluding that passive smoking has no effect, comparing tobacco industry affiliation with no tobacco industry affiliation? (This is, of course, the unadjusted odds ratio).

➕ 17.6.4   What is the corresponding relative risk?

❶➕ 17.6.5   Why are these two estimates quite different and what does this show about the interpretation of odds ratios?

17.7   The relationship between angina pectoris and plasma concentration of vitamins A, C and E was examined in a case–control study of 110 cases of angina and 394 controls. Plasma vitamin E remained independently related to the risk of angina after adjusting for age, smoking habit, blood pressure, lipids and relative weight. The adjusted odds ratio for angina for patients below the lowest and above the highest quintiles of vitamin E concentration was 2.98 (95% CI 1.07 to 6.70; $P = 0.02$). The authors concluded that some populations with a high incidence of coronary heart disease may benefit from diets rich in vitamin E (Riemersma *et al.* 1991).

➕ 17.7.1   What is meant by 'adjusted odds ratio of 2.98'? What method could be used to calculate it ?

➕ 17.7.2   How would you interpret this odds ratio?

➕ 17.7.3   Comment on the authors' conclusions.

17.8   In a prospective cohort study, subjects recruited between 1971 and 1974 had a standard dental examination. They were then followed for a median time of 14 years, and all deaths noted. Survival analysis using Cox proportional hazards regression was used to analyse the data. The crude relative risk of death from CHD in subjects with no teeth compared to subjects with no dental disease was 4.58. After adjustment for 13 potential risk factors, including blood pressure, serum cholesterol and cigarette smoking, the hazard ratio was 1.23 (95% CI 1.05 to 1.44) (De Stefano *et al.* 1993).

➕ 17.8.1   Why was survival analysis used in this study? What assumption is made by the Cox method?

ANSWERS

17.6.3   The odds ratio is calculated as the ratio of cross-products, odds ratio = $29 \times 65/(2 \times 10) = 94$ (*Intro* §13.7).

17.6.4   Risk of reporting no effect if tobacco industry affiliation = $29/31 = 0.94$. Risk of reporting no effect if no tobacco industry affiliation = $10/75 = 0.13$. Relative risk = $0.94/0.13 = 7$ (*Intro* §8.6).

17.6.5   The odds ratio is only a good estimate of the relative risk if the condition of interest is rare. Here, we are interested in the risk of reporting no harmful effects of passive smoking and this is not rare since about one-third ($39/106$) of reviews report no effects. In this study we can calculate the unadjusted relative risk directly and so we can compare the two estimates. We see that the unadjusted odds ratio (94) is much higher than the relative risk (7) (*Intro* §13.7).

17.7.1   This is the ratio of the odds of angina in those below the lowest and above the highest quintiles of vitamin E. The adjusted odds ratio expresses the association between angina and vitamin E after taking into account other measured variables which may be related to angina and vitamin E. It could be calculated using logistic regression because the outcome is dichotomous (angina, yes/no) and there are several possible predictor variables which need to be taken into account (*Intro* §13.7, 17.8).

17.7.2   Since angina is a relatively rare condition, the odds ratio from this case–control study is a reasonable estimate of the true relative risk. Hence we estimate that patients with low vitamin E levels have three times the risk of angina of patients with high vitamin E levels (*Intro* §13.7, 17.8).

17.7.3   The authors appear to have assumed that low vitamin E levels precede angina and so suggest that increasing vitamin E might reduce the risk. However, this is a case–control study and so we cannot say from this data that the relationship is this way round. It may be that low vitamin E is a by-product of angina or it may be that both are related to some other cause. The confidence interval is quite wide and the added risk may be quite small.

17.8.1   Subjects were recruited over several years, so some were observed for a longer period than others. Thus some subjects who had not yet died may have been observed for shorter periods than others who had died. Such observations are called 'censored'. Survival analysis deals with this problem. It also allows us to use data from subjects who died from other causes, who were at risk of CHD while they were alive, i.e. treating them as censored. The assumption is that for each factor considered (e.g. smoking) the instantaneous relative risk of dying, the hazard ratio, is the same throughout the study. This is the proportional hazards model (*Intro* §17.9).

QUESTIONS

● 17.8.2 Why might adjustment for risk factors have reduced the relative risk?

●● 17.8.3 What can we conclude about the possibility that the relationship between dental disease and CHD is causal?

17.9 An international randomized double-blind controlled trial compared combinations of zidovudine (AZT) plus didanosine (ddl) or zalcitabine (ddC) with AZT alone in 3 207 HIV-infected individuals. The authors reported that 'for analyses of adverse events, follow-up was censored at 30 days after stopping trial treatment'. Overall the study found that AZT in combination with ddl or ddC prolonged life and delayed disease progression compared with AZT alone. Hazard ratios for death were 0.67 (95% CI 0.56 to 0.80) for AZT+ddl versus AZT alone, 0.79 (95% CI 0.66 to 0.94) for AZT+ddC versus AZT alone and 0.85 (95% CI 0.70 to 1.02) for AZT+ddl versus AZT+ddC (Anonymous 1996).

● 17.9.1 Explain what is meant by 'censored' here.

● 17.9.2 What method could be used to compare survival in the three treatment groups when many patients are still alive?

● 17.9.3 What is meant by a hazard ratio and how would you interpret those here?

ANSWERS

17.8.2   We would have a relationship between toothlessness and CHD if both were related to some other confounding risk factor, such as diet. If poor diet led to toothlessness and to CHD, toothlessness and CHD would be related. Adjustment for this risk factor would then remove that component of the relationship due to the effect of the factor on each condition.

17.8.3   The relationship may not disappear completely because of measurement error in the risk factor. As most of the relationship vanished after adjustment, it is quite possible that adjustment for more risk factors and better measurement of the risk factors would remove the hazard ratio altogether. There is only weak evidence for the existence of a raised risk when other risk factors are taken into account, hence there is little evidence of causality.

17.9.1   The patients were followed up initially for 30 days after treatment ended. The outcome of interest was the occurrence of an adverse event. Adverse events occurring after 30 days are ignored. Thus, the observations are censored at 30 days (*Intro* §15.6).

17.9.2   For the analysis of time to death, observations are censored if the subject is still alive at the time of the analysis. Cox regression can be used to compare survival in several groups when some observations are censored. The method allows the data for all individuals to be used in the analysis until they die or are censored. Alternatively, the log-rank test could be used to compare survival in the three groups. Unlike Cox regression, this method would only give a P value and would not give an estimate of the size of effect (*Intro* §17.9).

17.9.3   The hazard ratio is the ratio of risk of death in the two respective groups at any given point in time. Hence, the ratio 0.67 shows that patients on the combination of drugs AZT+ddI had 0.67 of the risk of death of those on AZT alone. Similarly, patients taking AZT+ddC had 0.70 of the risk of death of those on AZT alone. Both of these hazard ratios are significant because the 95% CIs exclude the null value, 1.0. There is no significant difference in survival between the two combination drugs, since the 95% CI includes 1.0, although it seems that ddI may be better than ddC as the hazard ratio is 0.85 and may be as low as 0.70 (lower limit of CI) (*Intro* §15.6, 17.9).

QUESTIONS

17.10   In a study of the possible effects of passive smoking on birthweight (Peacock *et al.* 1998), the findings were combined with those of other studies in a meta-analysis. Wherever possible the difference was adjusted for other factors which might influence birthweight. The following table shows the estimated differences between the mean birthweights for non-smoking mothers not exposed to the cigarette smoke of others, and the mean birthweights for mothers who were passive smokers:

Study	n	Difference	(95% CI)
Rubin *et al.* (1986)	500	120 g per 20 cigarettes/day	
Martin and Bracken (1986)	2 473	24 g	(−13 to 60)
Haddow *et al.* (1988)	1 231	108 g	
Lazzaroni *et al.* (1990)	647	38 g	(−31 to 107)
Ogawa *et al.* (1991)	5 336	11 g	(−11 to 32)
Mathai *et al.* (1992)	994	63 g	(12 to 114)
Zhang and Radcliffe (1993)	1 785	30 g	(−7 to 66)
Martinez *et al.* (1994)	907	34 g per 10 cigarettes/day	(5 to 63)
Mainous and Hueston (1994)	1 173	84 g	(15 to 153)
Eskenazi *et al.* (1995)	2 243	45 g	(−36 to 125)
Peacock *et al.* (1998)	818	6.7 g	(−84 to 97)

For the meta-analysis, confidence intervals and standard errors for the studies of Rubin *et al.* and Haddow *et al.* were estimated from other data.

17.10.1   Why can publication bias be a problem in meta-analysis? How can a simple graphical method be used to investigate this?

17.10.2   Is publication bias likely to be a problem in this study?

17.10.3   Most studies estimated the difference between non-smokers exposed and non-smokers unexposed to passive smoke. Two gave the difference per 10 or 20 cigarettes per day smoked passively. What could the authors of the meta-analysis do about this?

ANSWERS

17.10.1 Publication bias is the process by which studies that report positive results are more likely to be published and published more prominently than studies that report negative results (*Intro* §17.11). A useful graphical check is the funnel plot, where we plot the magnitude of the effect against sample size. In the following figure, the left-hand plot shows a simulated data set of 30 studies where the true mean is 0, standard deviation 1, and the difference between two equal groups is plotted against total sample size. The curves are limits within which 95% of studies should lie:

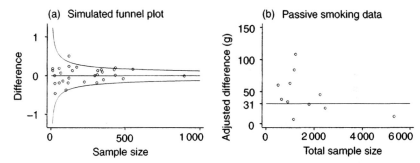

(a) Simulated funnel plot   (b) Passive smoking data

The right-hand plot shows the funnel plot for the passive smoking data. 31 g is the meta-analysis estimate of the difference. There appears to be a lack of small studies with small or negative differences. The bottom of the funnel is missing.

17.10.2 Publication bias is likely to be a problem here. There have been many studies of birthweight which have collected data on smoking by the parents. Some of these may not have analysed for passive smoking, others may have analysed for it but either not published it at all or published it with little prominence, as many potential risk factors would be considered. In these studies, low prominence is more likely if the difference is small, negative, or not significant. Hence, publication bias might be expected. The funnel plot shows a lack of studies in small sample, negative results end, where they would be expected if the meta-analysis estimate is correct. Hence we may be missing studies which would lower the overall effect.

17.10.3 We had to find some way to treat the estimates as equivalent. We decided to convert both rates to grams per 10 cigarettes per day. A pack of 20 cigarettes per day is typical of a smoker's consumption and we might suppose that the partner of a smoker might spend half their waking time in the smoker's company. Thus, 10 cigarettes per day might plausibly be considered typical exposure.

QUESTIONS

The authors reported that one study has shown large effects that remained after adjustment for age, education, height, parity, sex and weight, although gestational age was not controlled for (Haddow *et al.* 1988). Otherwise, most of the studies have shown relatively small effects after adjusting for confounders. There was no evidence for statistical heterogeneity ($\chi^2 = 12.9$, 10 d.f., P = 0.23).

17.10.4 What is the purpose of this test and what does the result encourage us to do?

The pooled estimate of difference in mean birthweight between the unexposed and exposed women across 11 studies was 31 g (95% CI 19 to 44).

17.10.5 What can we conclude from this? How does the possible publication bias influence our conclusions?

The paper included a figure similar to the one below:

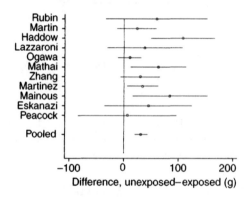

17.10.6 How might this figure be improved to better represent the data?

The authors concluded that 'Our data provide no support for a substantial effect of maternal passive smoking on birthweight ... The pooled estimate suggests that the effect of maternal passive smoking on birthweight is small ...'

17.10.7 Do you agree?

ANSWERS

17.10.4 In a meta-analysis, we assume that there is some overall common difference, which we want to estimate. We call this a fixed effects model. The test for heterogeneity is asking whether it is OK to assume that the population difference is the same for all studies. If so, we can estimate the difference ignoring any variation between studies, as in this case. If the test is significant, we cannot assume that there is a common difference which all the studies estimate. The population difference is not constant, but varies from study to study. We call this a random effects model. We could estimate the mean difference across a population of study populations. We would have to assume that these studies were carried out in a representative (i.e. can be treated as random) sample of all possible populations. The confidence interval using a random effects model would be much wider.

17.10.5 We can conclude that we estimate the effect of passive smoking on birthweight to be between 19 and 44 g. The effect of the possible publication bias would be to make these over-estimates. It seems fair to conclude that the effect of passive smoking, if any, on birthweight must be small.

17.10.6 We could make the points proportional to the total sample size for the comparison, to emphasize the large studies. We could also make the pooled estimate more distinctive, by using a lozenge shape:

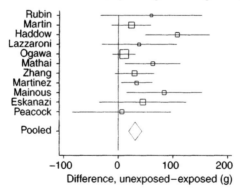

17.10.7 We hope you agree with our interpretation. The possible bias in the meta-analysis means that the estimate is, if anything, likely to be an over-estimate.

18
Determination of sample size

The methods in this chapter are usually taught only in postgraduate courses.

To determine the sample size for the estimation of a population mean or proportion, we must decide how precise we want the estimate to be. The width of the confidence interval depends on the sample size, so we decide what we want this to be and then calculate the sample size needed to achieve it.

For the comparison of means or proportions, as in a clinical trial or epidemiological study, we plan a significance test. The power of a test is the probability that the study will give a significant difference if the difference in the whole population is some chosen value. We might choose this value to be the smallest difference which would be clinically important, or the difference which two treatments might plausibly produce. The power depends on the sample size, so we can calculate the sample size required to achieve any given power of getting a significant difference in our study if the postulated population difference is correct.

For the comparison of two means, we need an estimate of the standard deviation of the outcome measurement. For the comparison of two proportions, we need an estimate of the proportion in the control group. To plan a study to detect a correlation we need only the size of the correlation we want to detect.

When the study subjects are in clusters, we need an estimate of the effect of clustering. This is usually an intraclass or intracluster correlation coefficient, and it can be hard to obtain. Using clusters may greatly increase the total sample required, particularly when large clusters are used.

QUESTIONS

18.1   In a general practice study, researchers planned to develop a risk scoring
system to detect patients with cervical cancer. The outcome of the study
was the sensitivity and specificity (proportion of cancer patients and
proportion of non-cancer patients that the test will correctly identify)
of the scoring system (Wilkinson *et al.* 1994).

What factors would the authors have taken account of in their sample
size calculations?

18.2   The following statement was made about the sample size for a randomized controlled trial comparing two treatments for relief of breathlessness: 'To detect a difference of 15% in relief of breathlessness rates at 4
months (from 65% to 80%) with significance level 0.05 and power 0.90
would require 400 patients to be randomized.' (MRC 1999).

18.2.1   Explain what is meant by 'significance level 0.05'.

18.2.2   Explain what is meant by 'power 0.90'.

18.2.3   In general terms, describe the effect on the required sample size if power
were reduced to 0.80.

18.2.4   In general terms, briefly describe the effect on the required sample size
if the difference to be detected was reduced to 10% (i.e. from 65% to
75%).

18.3   The following appeared in the report of a parallel group trial of two
cholesterol-lowering diets: 'In order to detect a change in plasma cholesterol concentration of 0.65 mmol/L with an α risk of 0.05 and a power
of 0.90 and allowing for a 30% withdrawal, we recruited 63 subjects.'
(Rivellese *et al.* 1994).

18.3.1   Explain what this statement means.

18.3.2   What additional information was needed to carry out the calculation?

ANSWERS

18.1   This study is estimating the sensitivity of the scoring system. To do this we need to have an estimate of the sensitivity anticipated and the precision required in terms of the width of the confidence interval. In addition, the confidence level must be set although this is usually taken as 95%. For example we might anticipate a sensitivity to be about 90% (0.90) and want to estimate this within about two percentage points (0.02). This would require the standard error to be 0.01 and hence, $n = 0.9 \times 0.1/0.01^2 = 900$ (*Intro* §18.2).

18.2.1 Significance level 0.05 means that if the null hypothesis were true and relief of breathlessness was the same for the two treatments in the population from which the patients came, then the probability of this trial (wrongly) giving a significant result would be 0.05 (*Intro* §9.4).

18.2.2 Power of 0.90 means that if the difference in breathlessness for patients given the two treatments was really 15 percentage points then the probability of this trial giving a significant result would be 0.90 (*Intro* §9.9).

18.2.3 If we reduce the power then the sample size required to detect the same difference would go down (*Intro* §18.3, 18.5).

18.2.4 If we reduce the size of difference to be detected then we will need more subjects (*Intro* §18.3, 18.5).

18.3.1 This is a calculation of sample size based on a significance test. α is the significance level, set in advance. It is almost always 0.05. The power is the probability of obtaining a significant difference, given that in the population there is a real difference. It depends on the magnitude of the difference. The authors have estimated the sample size required to give a probability of 0.90 that their study will produce a significant difference if the difference in the population is 0.65 mmol/L. Because they expect some subjects to drop-out of the trial, they have increased the sample size proportionately (*Intro* §18.3).

18.3.2 They need an estimate of the standard deviation of the cholesterol concentration (*Intro* §18.4).

QUESTIONS

18.4   A randomized trial was done on surgery for bile duct stones in patients who were at high risk of perioperative death. Keyhole surgery was compared to open surgery. The authors reported that 'the sample size was calculated according to expected decrease in mortality. On the assumption that mortality rate following surgical treatment of bileduct stones in elderly or high risk patients is 15%, the minimum number of patients required to demonstrate a reduction to 1% with keyhole surgery is 48 per group (alpha error 0.05, beta error 0.1).' (Targarona *et al.* 1996a).

18.4.1   In the calculation of sample size, what was the primary endpoint and what was the size of difference expected?

18.4.2   Does this sound a plausible difference in mortality to expect?

18.4.3   Could methods based on the Normal distribution used to calculate sample size for comparing two proportions work with such small numbers?

The study reported no differences in morbidity or mortality between the groups (mortality: keyhole surgery = 6%, open surgery = 4%, P = 0.5) and also no differences for 8 other endpoints but reported significant differences for 4 endpoints: length of stay (worse in open surgery group), recurrent biliary symptoms, readmission for biliary symptoms and cholecystectomy (worse in keyhole group). The study concluded that open surgery is to be recommended in preference to keyhole surgery in these patients.

18.4.4   In view of these results, what is the problem with the sample size calculation?

Subsequent correspondence (Peacock 1996, Targarona 1996b) about the paper indicated that the sample size calculation had in fact been done assuming that a one-tailed analysis was to be used.

18.4.5   What are the consequences of this approach? Do you think it is right?

18.4.6   How many comparisons appear to have been done altogether? What are the possible consequences of testing multiple endpoints?

18.4.7   If the tests had been one-tailed as suggested, is it possible to have a significant difference in favour of open surgery?

18.4.8   What did the authors conclude? How does this compare with the original aim of the study? Do you agree with the conclusions?

ANSWERS

18.4.1   The primary endpoint was mortality and the difference expected was 15% (open surgery) to 1% (keyhole surgery).

18.4.2   This is a huge difference in mortality rates. Differences of this magnitude in clinical trials are very unusual.

18.4.3   No, with a mortality rate of 1% in the keyhole surgery group and 48 subjects randomized, we would only expect 0.48 of a death and so methods based on the Normal distribution would be invalid (*Intro* §18.5).

18.4.4   The sample size calculations appear to have been based on an unrealistic difference—14 percentage points where in fact a difference of two percentage points was observed. Hence, the study is underpowered. There are also far fewer deaths in the open surgery group than were anticipated, which further reduces the power of the study.

18.4.5   A one-tailed analysis would test for differences in one direction only, here since it was expected that keyhole surgery would do better, any difference in the other direction would be ignored, however large. In other words if keyhole surgery did worse than open surgery, this could not be significant. This is not a reasonable approach because differences could clearly happen in either direction and we would want to know about any such differences. The effect on the sample size calculations is to reduce the required sample size compared to that required for a two-tailed test of the same power (*Intro* §9.5, 18.3).

18.4.6   It seems that 13 endpoints were tested, of which four were significant, one in favour of keyhole surgery and three in favour of open surgery. None of the significant endpoints had been the original primary outcome. When several endpoints are tested, the risk of a type I error is increased and so spurious significant results may be found (*Intro* §9.10).

18.4.7   No, if the tests had all been truly one-tailed, only differences in favour of keyhole surgery could be significant (*Intro* §9.5).

18.4.8   They concluded that open surgery was preferable to keyhole surgery in high risk patients because recurrent biliary symptoms were more common among the keyhole surgery group. This was not stated as the primary outcome, which was mortality and which showed no significant difference. The difference for biliary symptoms could be explained by chance (assuming a two-tailed test). If a one-tailed approach was really used then this could not be significant. We do not therefore agree with the authors' conclusions (*Intro* §9.5).

In view of these points and the one-tailed calculations, we think that this study was not adequately powered to investigate differences in mortality between the groups. A larger study, possibly multi-centre, would be needed to provide a clear answer to the question, is open surgery to be preferred to keyhole surgery.

QUESTIONS

18.5   To evaluate the effectiveness of an educational intervention in adolescent
health, general practitioners were randomized to receive the education or
to act as controls (Sanci *et al.* 2000). Consenting doctors were grouped
into eight geographical clusters by practice location to minimize contamination and to maximize efficiency of the delivery of the intervention.
Clusters of similar size were randomized by an independent researcher
to intervention or control groups. The intervention doctors in a cluster
were trained together. Questionnaires completed by the general practitioners were used to measure their knowledge, skill, and self-perceived
competency, satisfaction with the programme, and self-reported change
in practice. Sample size estimation was based on the minimum desirable
change in knowledge score. To detect an effect size difference of 0.67 in
a simple random sample with a power of 80% and significance level of
5%, 74 subjects were required. This figure was inflated to 148 to allow
for randomization by cluster (ICC = 0.05) and 20% attrition.

⊕ 18.5.1   What do they mean by 'effect size'?

⊕ 18.5.2   Why was the calculated sample size inflated to allow for randomization
by cluster?

⊕ 18.5.3   What is meant by 'ICC = 0.05'?

⊕ 18.5.4   Why was the calculated sample size inflated to allow for attrition?

ANSWERS

18.5.1   Effect size is the difference between the two treatment groups measured in standard deviations of the score.

18.5.2   The doctors in the same geographical group are being taught together. They may influence one another directly or may influence the teaching given. They also experience the same local conditions. As a result, the members of a group will be more like one another than they will be like members of other groups. They are not independent. We therefore need to take the clustering into account in the analysis, and this increases the size of difference which we can detect. We increase the sample size to compensate for this (*Intro* §18.8).

18.5.3   This is the intracluster or intraclass correlation coefficient, the correlation which we would get if we took pairs of subjects from each cluster. The hypothesised value of 0.05 is typical for such trials and was close to what was actually found after data had been collected (*Intro* §11.13, 18.8). Although such correlations may appear small, when clusters are large they may have a big effect.

18.5.4   It is inevitable that some participants will drop out in such a trial and will not provide data. Increasing the sample size ensures that there will be enough subjects completing the trial to achieve the planned power. In fact, 139 doctors were randomized and 108 actually took part, 22% dropout!

19
General questions

In this chapter there is no particular theme or body of material to be covered. Instead, we look at several research papers from start to finish. We have not attempted to reproduce the papers in full but have précised the key points. Many issues of study design, analysis and interpretation are revised.

We are grateful to the authors of the five papers in this chapter for agreeing that we could make extensive quotations from their work.

QUESTIONS

19.1   Birch *et al.* (1998) studied alcohol and drug use among junior hospital doctors. The sample were junior house officers (residents) in 18 National Health Service (NHS) Trust hospitals in the north-east of England. The authors contacted 114 house officers 1 year after graduation from Newcastle University and 90 agreed to participate. Anonymous information was obtained by a self-completed questionnaire, administered on site. The questionnaire asked about alcohol and drug consumption, anxiety and depression, and job satisfaction.

19.1.1   Which of the following terms do you think best describes the study, and why: case report, case series, case–control study, clinical trial, cohort study, cross-sectional study? Why is this design appropriate here?

19.1.2   Give two possible sources of bias in this sample as a sample of junior house officers in the UK.

19.1.3   What is the advantage of an anonymous questionnaire in this study?

Reported alcohol consumption (units/week) is shown in the table.

	Men $n = 39$	Women $n = 51$	Total $n = 90$
Mean (SD)	28.9 (20.1)	19.9 (13.5)	23.7 (17.2)
Median (range)	24.5 (1–84)	16.5 (1–60)	21 (1–84)
No alcohol	3 (7.7%)	3 (5.9%)	6 (6.7%)

The anxiety, depression and job satisfaction scores were:

	Men	Women	Total
Anxiety score	$n = 39$	$n = 50$	$n = 89$
Mean (SD)	5.4 (3.0)	6.8 (3.6)	6.2 (3.4)
Range	1–13	0–15	0–15
HAD Depression score	$n = 39$	$n = 50$	$n = 89$
Mean (SD)	2.5 (3.0)	3.2 (2.7)	2.9 (2.8)
Range	0–15	0–11	0–15
Job satisfaction score	$n = 39$	$n = 51$	$n = 90$
Mean (SD)	80.8 (15.8)	76.0 (14.8)	78.1 (15.3)
Range (median)	47–117 (80)	48–110 (76)	47–117 (78)

19.1.4   Percentages have been given to one decimal place, e.g. of 39 men the number who drank no alcohol was three, presented as 7.7%. Is this precision necessary or justified?

ANSWERS

19.1.1 This is a cross-sectional study. A single group of subjects is studied at one point in time. It is appropriate here because this is an attempt to do two things: to estimate the drinking and similar habits, psychological state, and work stress of junior house officers, and to see whether these are related. Thus everything is at the same time. Also, none of the conditions studied could be considered rare (*Intro* §3.6).

19.1.2 There are several possible biases: they were working in hospitals in the north-east of England only; drinking and drugging habits may be different elsewhere. They were from the University of Newcastle only; doctors from other medical schools were excluded and doctors' drinking may be related to their place of education. They were from 1 year of student enrolment only; doctors from other years of enrolment at Newcastle were excluded. Some doctors refused to take part; their alcohol consumption may be different. Biases of this sort are inevitable, as it would be very difficult to draw a truly representative sample of junior house officers, and there are bound to be some refusals (*Intro* §3.3, 3.5).

19.1.3 They did not want respondents to underestimate their drinking. They might do this if they thought their individual answers might become known to the researchers (*Intro* §3.9).

19.1.4 The percentages on either side of 7.7% are $2/39 = 5.1\%$ and $4/39 = 10.3\%$. Presenting these as 5%, 8%, and 10% is surely precise enough. They do not need a decimal place to differentiate these from the frequencies, as they include a % sign. The decimal place implies spurious precision (*Intro* §5.2).

QUESTIONS

19.1.5   Why can we deduce that the distribution of the HAD depression scale in these doctors is positively skew? What leads us the think that the distribution of the job satisfaction score is symmetrical?

More than 35% of men and 19% of women were currently using cannabis, with over 11% taking it regularly (weekly or monthly). Current use of other illegal drugs was reported by 13% of men and 10% of women. On the hospital anxiety and depression scale, 21% of men and 45% of women had anxiety scores of 8 or more, indicating possible pathological anxiety. Job satisfaction scores suggested some were dissatisfied with their job. Fifty-eight percent of men and 51% of women reported sleeping on average 7–8 hours per night whilst 42% and 49% slept 5–6 hours per night. Eight percent of men and 18% of women complained of difficulty getting to sleep and 23% and 53% were slow to become fully awake. Significant correlations were found between job satisfaction and anxiety scores ($r = -0.246$; P $= 0.02$) and between job satisfaction and depression ($r = -0.363$; P $= 0.001$), but not between alcohol or drug use and anxiety or occupational stress. The authors concluded that most of the house officers surveyed drink excessive amounts of alcohol; many use cannabis and take other illicit drugs. High scores for anxiety and mental ill-health were related to work pressures, but unrelated to the use of alcohol or illicit drugs. It is unlikely that these lifestyles apply only to house officers in the north east of England.

19.1.6   What does '$r = -0.246$' tell us about the relationship between job satisfaction score and anxiety?

19.1.7   What does P $= 0.001$ tell us about the relationship between job satisfaction score and depression score? Do you think the P value is valid?

19.1.8   What are the conclusions of the study and are they supported by the data?

19.2   Hobbs *et al.* (1996) carried out a study of psychological debriefing of people who had been in road traffic accidents. Those who agreed to the study were allocated using a table of random numbers to either an intervention or a non-intervention group. The intervention was an hour's debriefing combining a review of the event, encouragement of emotional expression, and promotion of cognitive processing of the experience. Advice was provided about common emotional reactions, the value of talking about the experience, and return to normal road travel. Both groups received an information leaflet consolidating this advice and encouraging the support of family and friends. Both groups were reassessed by interview and self-report questionnaires after four months.

19.2.1   What kind of study is this?

ANSWERS

19.1.5 For the depression scale, the standard deviation is greater than the mean, so if the distribution were symmetrical or negatively skew, it would have negative values, which are impossible. Also, the mean is near to the lower end of the range. For the job satisfaction scale, the median and the mean are almost equal. The median is also close to the middle of the range. Both these features suggest a symmetrical distribution (*Intro* §4.6, 4.8).

19.1.6 The coefficient is negative so job satisfaction score is higher in doctors with lower anxiety. The magnitude is small, so the relationship is weak (*Intro* §11.9).

19.1.7 P is much less than 0.05, so the relationship is significant. There is evidence that there is a relationship in the population. For the P value to be valid at least one variable should be from a Normal distribution. Depression score is skew, but job satisfaction score is symmetrical and so is likely to be approximately Normal, making the P value valid (*Intro* §9.3, 11.10).

19.1.8 The conclusions are that junior house officers have high levels of alcohol consumption and drug use and high anxiety scores. This is quite reasonable. It is implausible that only doctors from Newcastle have these characteristics, even though the estimates may be biased (*Intro* §3.5). The authors also say that the high anxiety scores are unrelated to alcohol or drug use. This is an interpretation of 'not significant' as meaning no relationship. An estimate of the correlation coefficient and its confidence interval would be helpful.

19.2.1 This is a randomized controlled clinical trial (*Intro* §2.2).

QUESTIONS

Despite intensive efforts, follow-up data were not obtained from 22% (16/54) of the intervention group and 6% (3/52) of controls. (The authors did not present a significant test for this difference, but it is significant, $\chi^2 = 5.9$, d.f. = 1, P = 0.02.) Non-respondents were reported not to differ on baseline characteristics.

19.2.2 Suggest two explanations for the different response rates in the two groups.

19.2.3 To what problems might this difference in response rates lead?

These were some of the results for the respondents (high scores mean high distress, etc.):

	Intervention ($n = 42$)	Non-intervention ($n = 49$)
Mean (SD) emotional distress score	0.62 (0.78)	0.38 (0.43)
Mean (SD) score on impact of events scale	15.97 (15.32)	12.87 (14.22)
No with distressing intrusive memories	9 (21%)	5 (10%)
Mean (SD) travel anxiety score	1.8 (1.68)	1.6 (1.7)
No with travel anxiety	18 (43%)	16 (33%)

19.2.4 What can be deduced about the distributions of the scores?

19.2.5 What tests of significance could be used to compare them?

From the table, we can see that the intervention group did worse on all the outcomes given. In addition, neither group showed a significant reduction in specific post-traumatic symptoms, mood disorder, anxiety, interview ratings of intrusive thoughts or travel anxiety, or clinical diagnosis of post-traumatic stress disorder or phobic anxiety. The intervention group had a worse outcome (P < 0.05) on two sub-scales of the brief symptom inventory, however, and a (non-significantly) poorer outcome in terms of emotional distress.

19.2.6 In the light of these results, which possible explanation for the different response rates in the two groups do you think is more plausible?

The authors concluded that despite the small numbers and lack of complete follow-up data, the findings are clinically convincing. Psychiatric morbidity was substantial four months after injury, with no evidence that debriefing had helped—and, indeed, indications that it might have been disadvantageous.

19.2.7 Are these conclusions supported by the brief summary of the results given here?

ANSWERS

19.2.2   The authors are right to draw attention to the problem of follow-up. It may be that patients who had received debriefing had recovered from the trauma so well that they had no further interest in the project. It may also be that they had recovered so poorly that they could not bear to discuss it again.

19.2.3   The groups may no longer be comparable. Some loss of subjects is to be expected in clinical trials and these researchers have achieved a high overall response rate (86%). As responders and non-responders do not differ significantly on baseline characteristics the respondents should be a reasonable sample of the whole study group. However, the non-response may be a treatment effect, where debriefing made the patients less likely to wish to respond to follow-up. We must treat any comparison with great caution.

19.2.4   The scores all have a standard deviation approximately equal to the mean. Such scores do not usually allow negative values. They cannot have symmetrical distributions, as if they did there would be observations less than mean minus two standard deviations. They must be positively skew (*Intro* §4.8).

19.2.5   We are comparing two independent groups. If we want to treat the scores as interval data, we could try a log transformation and a two sample t test. Otherwise, we could use a Mann–Whitney U test (*Intro* §14.3).

19.2.6   The explanation that refusers had recovered so poorly that they could not bear to discuss it again seems the more plausible to us. The responders in the intervention group had more morbidity than the responders in the non-intervention group. We cannot, of course, know the truth about why people refuse to respond, and there may be many other possible explanations.

19.2.7   Yes, a lot of subjects still had distressing memories and travel anxiety. There is no evidence from the responders that the intervention had reduced this and if anything the intervention group fared worse. The differential non-response suggests the possibility of an even bigger difference.

QUESTIONS

19.3   Mann *et al.* (1993) studied subsequent mortality in drunken drivers. The sample consisted of all individuals convicted of a second drinking and driving offence in two Ontario cities between 1973 and late 1978. These individuals were assigned to attend brief educational programmes and were identified based on programme records. A total of 639 individuals (25 females and 614 males) were identified. The mean age of the sample at programme entry was 35.6 years (SD = 11.2, range = 17–67).

Data collection proceeded in several stages. First, programme records were searched to identify participants and other relevant information. Second, the Ministry of Transportation provided current address information for those individuals identified. Third, efforts to contact each individual either by mail or telephone were made; direct contact was made with roughly 40% of the initial sample. The fourth stage consisted of additional review of Ministry of Transportation records for further information on that portion of the sample for which contact could not be made, and attempts to contact individuals for whom revised address information was available.

Several individuals were identified as deceased based on initial programme records, Ministry of Transportation records, or a relative's report. Ontario death records were searched for cause of death information for people thus identified; as well, these records were searched for individuals who could not be located or contacted. The death record search involved the years 1973–1986 inclusive. A total of 53 deaths were thus identified; Ontario death records were located for 43 of these individuals. In view of the probability that an unknown number of the individuals who could not be located had moved and subsequently died outside of the province, this total was thought likely to be an underestimate. Ontario vital statistics for the years of follow-up were used to calculate expected mortality.

19.3.1   Which of the following terms do you think best describes the study, and why: case report, case series, cross-sectional study, cohort study, case–control study, clinical trial?

19.3.2   Why is this method appropriate here?

Among males, 51 deaths were observed and 30.23 were expected. Thus, the Standardized Mortality Ratio (SMR) for the male drinking drivers was 1.7 when compared to that of the general Ontario population; that is, they were 70% more likely to die over the follow-up period.

19.3.3   What is an SMR and why is this method used here?

19.3.4   Is the explanation of what an SMR of 1.7 means given here correct?

ANSWERS

19.3.1   This is best described as a cohort study, because a group of people is identified and then followed over time until the event of interest (death) occurs. It differs from most cohort designs in that the cohort all have the risk factor (drinking and driving) and they are compared to the general population (*Intro* §3.7).

19.3.2   If we were to start with the outcome, death, there would be great problems in ascertainment of who was a drinking driver. If we start with the risk factor (drinking and driving) we need to follow people over time to get sufficient deaths.

19.3.3   The SMR is found by dividing the number of deaths observed among the drinking drivers by the number of deaths which we would expect if the drinking drivers had the same mortality rates at each age as the population of Ontario. It is used because the age distribution is not the same in the drivers and the Ontario population. This could lead to a difference in the number of deaths in the two groups, because older people have much greater risks of death than young people. Here the drivers tend to be young and middle aged adults, with few elderly people. We therefore adjust for age (*Intro* §16.3). Note that this calculation was for males only. There were not enough females in the sample.

19.3.4   Yes, but it applies only to a population with the drivers' age distribution. Drinking drivers experienced 1.7 times the number of deaths of a group of the general Ontario population with the same age distribution. Hence their probability of death was 0.7 or 70% greater than in such a group from the general population. The excess risk of death will not necessarily be the same at each age (*Intro* §16.3).

QUESTIONS

The probability of witnessing the observed or greater number of deaths, given the expected number of deaths, was 0.000 5. This was calculated based on the Poisson probability distribution.

19.3.5   Why was the Poisson probability distribution used?

19.3.6   Is this significance test one-sided or two-sided? How does the likely failure to identify all the deaths make their approach correct?

Among females, two deaths were observed and 0.49 were expected, for a SMR of 4.07. The probability of observing this number of deaths or more among the females was 0.088. Because of the small number of females in the sample, no further analysis of their mortality was performed.

19.3.7   This SMR is not significant. Can we conclude that there is no excess mortality among women drinking drivers?

Male mortality was analysed by age groups:

Age group	Observed	Expected	SMR	P of observed or greater no. of deaths
15–34	7	2.72	2.57	0.0214
35–54	24	12.17	1.97	0.0018
55–79	20	15.34	1.30	0.144

19.3.8   In this table, what can be concluded from each of the P values?

19.3.9   The authors may not have identified all the deaths. What effects might this have on the study?

The male deaths were also broken down by cause:

Cause	Observed	Expected	SMR	P
Cancer of the lung	5	2.61	1.91	0.1
Ischaemic heart disease	9	9.50	0.95	0.6
Cerebrovascular disease	4	1.21	3.31	0.03
Chronic liver disease and cirrhosis	7	1.16	6.02	0.0003
Accidental and violent deaths	10	5.09	1.97	0.04
Motor vehicle accidents	3	1.37	2.19	0.2
Alcohol dependence syndrome	2	0.29	6.87	0.04
Other*	11			

*Includes reported deaths for which no death certificate could be found.

19.3.10   What is the difference between the presentation of the P values in the first and second tables? Which do you think is better?

19.3.11   Why should we not conclude that being a drinking driver causes people to die of cerebrovascular disease?

ANSWERS

19.3.5 This is the distribution followed by the number of events in a fixed time, where they happen randomly and independently. This will be the case unless they occur in a rapid epidemic or natural disaster. Such death counts are usually treated as following a Poisson distribution (*Intro* §6.7).

19.3.6 The test is one-sided, because they only include the probability of excess deaths, not the probability of fewer deaths than expected. If we find that there are fewer deaths among drinking drivers, this may be because drinking and driving is related to a lower risk of death, or it may be that we have not found all the deaths. Thus the null hypothesis is that the death rate as ascertained among drinking drivers is lower than or equal to that for the general population, a one-tailed test (*Intro* §9.5).

19.3.7 No. 'Not significant' does not mean there is no effect. We have merely failed to demonstrate that one exists (*Intro* §9.6).

19.3.8 For age group 15–34, there is evidence that the death rate was higher than expected. For age group 35–54, the evidence that the death rate was higher than expected is strong. For age group 55–79, the evidence is very weak and if we only had this age group we would not be able to draw any conclusions. We cannot conclude that there is no difference (*Intro* §9.4, 9.6).

19.3.9 We may underestimate the SMRs. We are comparing these deaths to the general population, where all deaths are known. Thus any excess risk of death may be underestimated by an unknown amount.

19.3.10 In their first table (Question 19.3.7) the authors gave P values to several significant figures, in the second table (Question 19.3.9) to only one significant figure. We do not think that much information is conveyed by the second and subsequent significant figures in a P value. Using only one significant figure makes the table easier to read, so we prefer the second approach.

19.3.11 This is an observational study and so we cannot be sure of causality. Death from cerebrovascular disease and drinking and driving may both be due to some other factor. In this paper strong arguments are given for thinking that both are the result of high alcohol consumption, i.e. that the driving may have nothing to do with it.

QUESTIONS

The authors note that several restrictions must be placed on interpretation of their results: the small sample size, subjects lost to follow-up, inability to find death certificates for nine individuals who were identified as deceased, possibility of bias in the selection of individuals referred by courts to the programme, bias in police detection practices.

Keeping these restrictions in mind, they note several very interesting findings in this work. Foremost is the finding that convicted second offenders experienced 70% greater mortality than expected over the follow-up interval. The cause-specific mortality clearly suggests the behavioural pattern leading to this excess mortality, i.e. alcohol abuse. The pattern of excess mortality corresponds remarkably closely to that observed in mortality studies of alcoholics. The largest increase in risk in the sample was from causes most strongly related to alcohol consumption (liver cirrhosis, alcohol dependence syndrome). As well, excess mortality from accidental and violent death and stroke was also found; alcohol abusers also are at increased risk from these causes.

One question that arises when drinking and driving counter-measures are considered is the extent to which convicted drinking drivers represent a problem-drinking or a problem-driving population. A substantial proportion of convicted drinking drivers have serious alcohol problems. Evidence for personality factors as precursors to drinking and driving behaviour highlight the potential usefulness of programmes aimed at reducing such factors as risk-taking and aggressiveness. On the other hand, there are similarities between personality correlates of drinking drivers and alcohol abusers. This study demonstrates a substantial agreement between patterns of excess mortality in drinking drivers and alcoholics and suggests that the alcohol problem is fundamental, at least in this sample of second offenders. However, the authors note that a lack of mortality data on other relevant groups (such as problem drivers without drinking problems) precludes a clear answer to the question.

19.3.12 The main conclusions of the study are that drinking drivers experience increased mortality and that this is the result of alcohol abuse, not problem driving. Are these conclusions supported by the data?

ANSWERS

19.3.12 Convicted second offenders experienced 70% increased mortality (SMR $= 1.7$, P $= 0.0005$). There is certainly an excess of deaths, whereas the bias of the study is in the opposite direction. The highest SMRs are for alcohol-related conditions (liver, alcohol dependence), not driving related conditions (motor vehicle accidents). Reference is made to other studies which show a similar pattern of mortality among alcohol abusers. As there is no similar study for mortality in non-drinking problem drivers, we cannot be sure.

QUESTIONS

19.4   Winters *et al.* (1997) carried out a single-blind randomized trial comparing physiotherapy, manipulation and corticosteroid injection for treating
shoulder complaints in general practice. The subjects were divided into
two diagnostic groups: a shoulder girdle group ($n = 58$) and a synovial
group ($n = 114$). Patients in the shoulder girdle group were randomized
to manipulation or physiotherapy, and patients in the synovial group
were randomized to corticosteroid injection, manipulation, or physiotherapy. Corticosteroid injections were given by the participating doctors immediately after randomization, 1 week later, and, if needed, after
a further 2 weeks. Manipulation was done by either the participating
general practitioners or physiotherapists. They were instructed in which
techniques to use. Physiotherapy was given twice a week by local physiotherapists. No mobilization techniques or manipulative techniques
were allowed, to keep the manipulation and physiotherapy regimes dis-
tinct. After treatment had started, the patients were asked to complete
a pain questionnaire each week. This gave a pain score, obtained by
rating seven aspects of pain, each from one to four, giving a total score
between 7 points (no pain) and 28 points (severe pain). They were also
asked to indicate if they felt cured or if they thought that the treatment
had failed. Follow-up physical examinations after randomization were
done by a physiotherapist who was not informed about the patients'
diagnosis and treatment.

19.4.1   This is described as a single-blind study. Who is blinded and why was
this done?

19.4.2   How easy would it be to break the blinding?

19.4.3   What might be the effects of the problems with blinding in this study?

The figure below shows the percentage of shoulder girdle patients still
with symptoms at different times after the start of the trial:

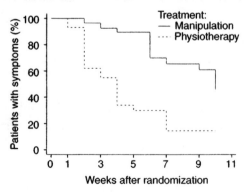

19.4.4   What kind of graph is this?

ANSWERS

19.4.1 The only person who was blinded to treatment was the physiotherapist who did the follow-up assessments. This was done so that the physiotherapist would not be biased in the assessments by wanting one treatment to succeed or believing that it should (*Intro* §2.9).

19.4.2 The patients know their treatment and may mention this to the physiotherapist. It would be quite easy for the blinding to be broken and difficult to maintain it.

19.4.3 The patients cannot be blinded to treatment and the knowledge of what the treatment is will be part of the treatment. Thus if a patient starts out with a preference for medical treatment, for example, this may influence the reports of pain, decreasing pain scores if on injection and increasing it if on other treatments. If the physiotherapist carrying out the follow-up knows the treatment, a bias, conscious or unconscious, in favour of physiotherapy, say, may influence the measurements. It is difficult to see any way round these problems (*Intro* §2.8).

19.4.4 These are Kaplan–Meier survival curves, showing the 'survival' in a symptomatic state (*Intro* §15.6).

QUESTIONS

19.4.5   With reference to the previous graph, the authors say that 'manipulation
         was superior to physiotherapy (P < 0.001)'. What does 'P < 0.001'
         mean?

⊕ 19.4.6   What method might be used to calculate it?

19.4.7   What can we conclude from this test?

The pain scores of patients in the shoulder girdle group, at randomization to treatment and at the end of treatment (when the patient left the
study or 11 weeks after randomization) were compared. The following
table shows the mean (SD) of the pain scores at each time:

	Manipulation ($n = 32$)	Physiotherapy ($n = 35$)
At randomization	14.8 (4.2)	14.4 (3.5)
At end of treatment	9.9 (3.5)[†]	12.0 (4.4) [†]

[†] Significant difference from pain score at randomization (P < 0.001)

19.4.8   In the above table, what methods could be used to calculate the P values
         and what would influence the choice?

19.4.9   Why is this not the most useful comparison which could be made? What
         comparison would have been more useful?

⊕ 19.4.10 For the synovial group, there were three treatment groups, analysed in
           the same way. What method could be used for a more useful comparison
           here?

For the synovial group, survival analysis of the symptomatic state
showed a significant difference between the treatment groups (P <
0.001). The corticosteroid injection group improved rapidly, while the
physiotherapy group improved slowly and the manipulation group did
only slightly better. At 5 weeks after randomization, 75% of patients
in the injection group were 'cured' compared with 20% in the physiotherapy group and 40% in the manipulation group. Drop-out because
of treatment failure was much lower in the injection group (17% (7/47))
than in the physiotherapy group (51% (18/35)) and manipulation group
(59% (19/32)).

19.4.11 What statistical method could be used to compare the frequency of
         drop-out due to treatment failure between the groups and why?

Some patients were reported to have been 'cured' before 11 weeks after
randomization. Among these patients, a recurrence of complaints by
week 11 was reported by 18% (7/39) of patients in the injection group,
13% (2/15) in the physiotherapy group, and 8% (1/13) in the manipulation group.

❗ 19.4.12 There are two problems, one of analysis and one of design, in testing
          the frequency of recurrence. What are they?

ANSWERS

19.4.5   This is the result of a significance test. It means that if there was
no difference in the effects of manipulation and physiotherapy in this
population of patients, the probability of a difference in a sample as
large as the difference observed here was less than 0.001.

19.4.6   It could be calculated using the log-rank test (*Intro* §9.3).

19.4.7   We can conclude that there is good evidence that patients receiving
manipulation do better than those receiving physiotherapy (*Intro* §9.4,
9.6).

19.4.8   The comparisons are of paired data, before and after for each patient.
The score can be treated like a measurement and a paired t test used. If
the distribution of the differences were not Normal, the Wilcoxon paired
test could be used instead. If the scores could not be treated as interval
measurements, the sign test could be used (*Intro* §14.4).

19.4.9   This test tells us that the patients in each group had lower mean pain
scores at the end of the treatment. It does not tell us whether one
treatment lowered pain more than did the other. A comparison between
the mean changes in the two groups, or between the mean final scores,
would be better. This could be done using a two sample t test or
a Mann–Whitney U test. What is the point in randomizing to get
comparable groups and then not comparing them? (*Intro3* §9.6). The
authors told us that they did compare the groups directly in a separate,
more extensive publication (Jan Winters, personal communication).

19.4.10 There are more than two groups, so we cannot use the two sample
t test. A one-way analysis of variance could be used, followed by a
multiple comparison procedure. The non-parametric alternative would
be the Kruskal–Wallis test (*Intro* §14.5).

19.4.11 We have the relationship between two categorical variables, treatment
and drop-out. We can construct a 3×2 contingency table and carry out
a chi-squared test. The test is highly significant, $\chi^2 = 19.4$, d.f. $= 2$,
$P = 0.0001$ (*Intro* §14.5, 13.1).

19.4.12 The analytical problem is that the numbers are too small for a chi-
squared test. As the total number with recurrences is 10 in three groups,
at least two of the expected frequencies must be less than 5 (as they
cannot be zero) (*Intro* §13.3). Fisher's exact test could be used if a
suitable program were available (*Intro* §13.4). The design problem, as
the authors noted in their discussion, is that the injection group, being
'cured' earlier, had more opportunity to recur.

QUESTIONS

The authors concluded that the results suggest that manipulation is to be preferred to physiotherapy for treating shoulder complaints originating from the shoulder girdle in general practice. They also conclude that injection is the most effective treatment for shoulder complaints originating from the synovial structures in general practice.

19.4.13 On the basis of the partial summary given here, do you think that these conclusions are reasonable?

Winters *et al.* (1999) followed up this trial by sending a questionnaire to all participants, between 2 and 3 years after treatment. They received 130 (76%) questionnaires that could be evaluated. The distribution of the patients' characteristics across the five treatment groups was similar to the original study.

19.4.14 Why is the response rate important and what does the distribution of patients characteristics tell us?

In the shoulder girdle group, 29/40 (73%) patients had experienced a shoulder complaint at some time since the earlier trial. Thirteen of the 22 (59%) patients in the physiotherapy group had current complaints, of whom 8 (62%) did not feel cured. (In these studies, feeling 'cured' was defined as disappearance of shoulder complaints or a decrease of shoulder complaints to such an extent that they were no longer inconvenient, did not need treatment, or no longer interfered with normal working.) In the manipulation group 6/18 (33%) patients had current complaints, of whom four did not feel cured. No significant differences were found between the two treatments. In the synovial group 47/90 (52%) patients had experienced a shoulder complaint at some time since the trial. No significant differences were found between the three treatment groups. The authors concluded that the positive results of both injection therapy and manipulation versus physiotherapy in the original trial seemed to be short-term effects.

19.4.15 Do you agree with the authors' conclusions from the follow-up study?

ANSWERS

19.4.13 The conclusions are reasonable. There is a significant treatment effect in each group. If there were an observer bias in favour of physiotherapy, it is not apparent in the results, although of course the observer may have been aware of the bias, leading to an attempt to correct it and a resulting bias in the other direction. The authors rightly emphasize that their results only apply to the general practice setting which they studied. The main caveat would be that some recurrences were observed and that a longer follow-up may have been informative.

19.4.14 If some patients provide no information, then the follow-up sample may not truly represent the original patients. Also, the groups may no longer be comparable. The similarity of patient characteristics across the group helps to reassure us that there is not a serious problem here. The response rate is quite high for a postal questionnaire.

19.4.15 As more than half of the patients had had further shoulder problems since the trial, the authors seem quite justified in concluding that the treatment benefits were not permanent for many patients. It is difficult to conclude that there were no treatment differences, as this depends on differences being not significant. 'Not significant' does not mean there was no difference (*Intro* §9.6). The difference between 59% and 33% is quite large, even if not significant. The sample is too small to detect differences between treatment groups unless they were large.

QUESTIONS

19.5   Spontaneous pneumothorax is the presence of air or gas in the pleural
space without known cause. Two treatments, simple aspiration and
intercostal tube drainage, were compared in a randomized controlled
trial (Harvey and Prescott 1994). Each treatment involves inserting
a tube to remove excess air, in simple aspiration the tube is removed
after air has been removed, in intercostal drainage it is left in place for
a while. Of the 35 patients allocated to simple aspiration, 7 were not
aspirated successfully and intercostal drainage was used. Some of the
patients pre-treatment data are shown in the table:

	Aspiration	Intercostal drain	P value
Age (years) mean (SD) (n)	34.6 (15.0) $(n = 35)$	34.6 (13.1) $(n = 38)$	0.8
Sex (M/F)	28/7	29/9	0.92
Height (m) mean (SD) (n)	1.79 (0.11) $(n = 32)$	1.76 (0.09) $(n = 3l)$	0.81
Weight (kg) mean (SD) (n)	64.8 (9.2) $(n = 31)$	63.6 (11.0) $(n = 37)$	0.65
Smoking history (pack years) mean (SD) (n)	8.09 (9.32) $(n = 34)$	7.94 (9.16) $(n = 38)$	0.95

19.5.1 What shape do you think the distribution of smoking history has?

19.5.2 What statistical method could be used for each of the tests given?

The following table shows the nature of the pneumothorax, before treatment:

Size of pneumothorax	Aspiration	Intercostal drain	P value
Small rim	3	1	0.054
Partial collapse	16	12	
Complete collapse	10	18	

19.5.3 What statistical method could be used to find the P value here?

19.5.4 What null hypotheses are being tested in this and the preceding table
(age to size of pneumothorax)? Are these useful things to test?

ANSWERS

19.5.1   The distribution must be skew to the right. This is obvious because the standard deviation is greater than the mean. A symmetrical distribution will have observations around mean minus two standard deviations or even less (*Intro* §4.8).

19.5.2   We have two small independent samples. For the measurements we could consider the two-sample t test, possibly with a transformation, or the Mann–Whitney U test. For each of them the standard deviations are similar in the two groups. The distribution of age is unknown, so we do not have enough information to say, height is well known to follow a Normal distribution so a t test could be used, weight may be positively skew and may require a transformation before a t test. Smoking is highly skew and is likely to have a group of zeros for non-smokers. Transformation may be difficult because of the zeros so the Mann–Whitney U test may be preferred. The yes-or-no variables could be compared by chi-squared test, comparison of two proportions or Fisher's exact test. The expected frequencies all exceed five, so any of these tests would do (*Intro* §14.2).

19.5.3   This is a 3×2 contingency table. The total for the first row is 4, so both expected frequencies will be considerably less than 5. We could combine rows 'small rim' and 'partial collapse' to give a 2×2 table. Alternatively, we could take the ordering of the rows into account and do a chi-squared test for trend or a similar method, which does not require such stringent conditions on the expected frequencies. We think that this is what the authors did (*Intro* §13.3, 13.8). Another possibility would be Fisher's exact test for a 3×2 table (*Intro3* §13.4) but this would not take the order into account.

19.5.4   The null hypothesis in each case is that there is no difference in the mean or proportion of this variable between aspiration and intercostal patients in the population from which they come. As they are randomized, the two groups come from the same population and these null hypotheses are true by definition. The tests are therefore superfluous.

QUESTIONS

Patients completed symptom score charts indicating the degree of pain experienced during drainage and throughout their hospital admission. Patients were reviewed at one and 12 months, and recurrence of pneumothorax or referral for thoracic surgery was recorded. The outcomes are shown in this table:

	Aspiration	Intercostal drain	P
% Predicted FEV1 after 1 month, mean (SD) (n)	94.5 (25.7) (n = 16)	97.3 (17.1) (n=20)	0.70
Pain score during procedure	0.9 (0.9) (n = 35)	1.1 (0.9) (n = 38)	0.33
Average daily pain score	0.7 (0.7) (n = 35)	1.5 (0.6) (n = 38)	0.001
Total pain score	2.7 (3.3) (n = 35)	6.7 (3.6) (n = 38)	0.001
Hospital stay (days)			
Mean (SD) (n)	3.2 (2.9) (n = 35)	5.3 (3.6) (n = 38)	0.005
Median	2	4.5	
Number having pleurectomy within 1 year	0 (n = 35)	7 (n = 38)	0.02
Number of recurrences	5 (n = 30)	10 (n = 35)	0.40

19.5.5   What statistical method could be used for each of the tests given?

19.5.6   Not all the patients in the first column of the table had a successful aspiration, seven actually had an intercostal drain. Why are they included with the patients who received successful aspiration?

19.5.7   Is this study blind? Does this have any implications for the interpretation of the results?

19.5.8   Why would confidence intervals be a more informative approach to the analysis?

The authors concluded that simple aspiration is a simple and safe procedure and should be the initial treatment of choice for patients with normal lungs who present with a spontaneous pneumothorax. Aspiration is less painful than intercostal drainage, leads to a shorter hospital stay, and reduces the need for pleurectomy with no increase in recurrence rate at 1 year.

19.5.9   Are the conclusions justified by the data?

ANSWERS

19.5.5 Again, we have two small independent samples. Except for FEV, the measurements all have highly skew distributions. For FEV we could consider the two sample t test. For the pain scores it is questionable whether we have an interval scale of measurement and so the Mann–Whitney U test may be preferable. Days in hospital is highly skew and discrete, because the observations will be whole numbers of days. It might be very difficult to transform because of this and again the Mann–Whitney U test may be preferable. Pleurectomy and recurrence are both dichotomous, so chi-squared or Fisher's exact test will be appropriate. For pleurectomy the expected frequencies will be small, so we need Fisher's exact test or a chi-squared test with Yates' correction (*Intro* §14.2).

19.5.6 They were allocated to aspiration, and are kept in that group to ensure that the two treatment groups are comparable apart from treatment. The analysis is by intention to treat (*Intro* §2.5).

19.5.7 It is not blind, as the patients and the doctors know what treatment is being given. This should make us a little cautious in interpreting the pain scores. Because of the lack of blindness, knowledge of treatment given must be regarded as part of the treatment (*Intro* §2.7, 2.8).

19.5.8 Confidence Intervals would show us the possible sizes of the differences, rather than simply indicate that differences exist or that they may not.

19.5.9 The conclusion is that simple aspiration leads to less pain and shorter hospital stay, reduces the need for pleurectomy and shows no increase in recurrence. This seems well supported by the data, although it would be better to say that we have not shown an excess in recurrence rather than showing no increase.

References

Abu-Arefeh, I. and Russell, G. (1994). Prevalence of headache and migraine in school-children. *British Medical Journal*, **309**, 765–9.

Ajayi, V., Miskelly, F.G., and Walton, I.G. (1995). The NHS and Community Care Act 1990: is it a success for elderly people? *British Medical Journal*, **310**, 439.

Alary, M., Joly, J.R., Moutquin, J.M., Mondor, M., Boucher, M., Fortier, A., Pinault, J.J., Paris, G., Carrier, S., Chamberland, H., *et al.* (1994). Randomised comparison of amoxycillin and erythromycin in treatment of genital chlamydial infection in pregnancy. *Lancet*, **344**, 1461–5.

Altmann, P., Dhanesha, U., Hamon, C., Cunningham, J., Blair, J., and Marsh, F. (1989). Disturbance of cerebral function by aluminium in haemodialysis patients without overt aluminium toxicity. *Lancet*, **2**, 7–12.

Anonymous (1990). GISSI-2: a factorial randomised trial of alteplase versus strep-tokinase and heparin versus no heparin among 12,490 patients with acute myocardial infarction. Gruppo Italiano per lo Studio della Sopravvivenza nell'Infarto Miocardico. *Lancet*, **336**, 65–71.

Anonymous (1991). Single dose cabergoline versus bromocriptine in inhibition of puer-peral lactation: randomised, double blind, multicentre study. European Multicentre Study Group for Cabergoline in Lactation Inhibition. *British Medical Journal*, **302**, 1367–71.

Anonymous (1996). Delta: a randomised double-blind controlled trial comparing com-binations of zidovudine plus didanosine or zalcitabine with zidovudine alone in HIV-infected individuals. Delta Coordinating Committee. *Lancet*, **348**, 283–91.

Appleby, L. (1991). Suicide during pregnancy and in the first postnatal year. *British Medical Journal*, **302**, 137–40.

Barnes, D.E. and Bero, L.A. (1998). Why review articles on the health effects of passive smoking reach different conclusions. *JAMA*, **279**, 1566–70.

Birch, D., Ashton, H., and Kamali, F. (1998). Alcohol, drinking, illicit drug use, and stress in junior house officers in north-east England. *Lancet*, **352**, 785–6.

Bisset, A.F. and Russell, D. (1994). Grommets, tonsillectomies, and deprivation in Scotland. *British Medical Journal*, **308**, 1129–32.

Blair, P.S., Fleming, P.J., Smith, I.J., Platt, M.W., Young, J., Nadin, P., Berry, P.J., and Golding, J. (1999). Babies sleeping with parents: case–control study of factors influencing the risk of the sudden infant death syndrome. *British Medical Journal*, **319**, 1457–61.

Bland, J.M., Bewley, B.R., and Banks, M.H. (1979). Cigarette smoking and children's respiratory symptoms: validity of questionnaire method. *Revue d'Epidemiologie et Sante Publique*, **27**, 69–76.

Bland, J.M. and Altman, D.G. (1995). Statistics Notes. Calculating correlation coefficients with repeated observations: Part 1, correlation within subjects. *British Medical Journal*, **310**, 446.

Bland, M. (2000a). Fatigue and psychological distress—statistics are improbable (letter). *British Medical Journal*, **320**, 515.

Bland, M. (2000b). *An Introduction to Medical Statistics* 3rd ed., Oxford Medical Publications, Oxford.

Bonnar, J. and Sheppard, B.L. (1996). Treatment of menorrhagia during menstruation: randomised controlled trial of ethamsylate, mefenamic acid, and tranexamic acid. *British Medical Journal*, **313**, 579–82.

Bosely, S. (1999). The lottery babies. *The Guardian*, London, 24 July, p.8.

Bridges, B.A., Cole, J., Arlett, C.F., Green, M.H., Waugh, A.P., Beare, D., Henshaw, D.L., and Last, R.D. (1991). Possible association between mutant frequency in peripheral lymphocytes and domestic radon concentrations. *Lancet*, **337**, 1187–9.

Bromwich, P., Cohen, J., Steward, I., and Walker, A. (1994). Decline in sperm counts: an artefact of changed reference range of 'normal'? *British Medical Journal*, **309**, 19–22.

Burker, E.J., Blumenthal, J.A., Feldman, M., Burnett, R., White, W., Smith, L.R., Croughwell, N., Schell, R., Newman, M., and Reves, J.G. (1995). Depression in male and female patients undergoing cardiac surgery. *British Journal of Clinical Psychology*, **34**, 119–28.

Campbell, M.J. and Gardner, M.J. (1989). Calculating confidence intervals for some non-parametric analyses. In Gardner M.J. and Altman D.G. (ed.) *Statistics with Confidence*, British Medical Journal, London.

Carbajal, R., Paupe, A., Hoenn, E., Lenclen, R., and Olivier-Martin, M. (1997). DAN: une echelle comportementale d'evaluation de la douleur aigue du nouveau-ne. *Archives de Pediatrie*, **4**, 623–8.

Carbajal, R., Chauvet, X., Couderc, S., and Olivier-Martin, M. (1999). Randomised trial of analgesic effects of sucrose, glucose, and pacifiers in term neonates. *British Medical Journal*, **319**, 1393–7.

Chalder, T. and Wessley, S.C. (2000). Fatigue and psychological distress—authors' reply. *British Medical Journal*, **320**, 515.

Chandna, S.M., Schulz, J., Lawrence, C., Greenwood, R.N., and Farrington, K. (1999). Is there a rationale for rationing chronic dialysis? A hospital based cohort study of factors affecting survival and morbidity. *British Medical Journal*, **318**, 217–23.

Churchill, D., Perry, I.J., and Beevers, D.G. (1997). Ambulatory blood pressure in pregnancy and fetal growth. *Lancet*, **349**, 7–10.

Clarke, K.W., Gray, D., Keating, N.A., and Hampton, J.R. (1994). Do women with acute myocardial infarction receive the same treatment as men? *British Medical Journal*, **309**, 563–6.

Cohen, D., Green, M., Block, C., Slepon, R., Ambar, R., Wasserman, S.S., and Levine, M.M. (1991). Reduction of transmission of shigellosis by control of houseflies (*Musca domestica*). *Lancet*, **337**, 993–7.

Cohen, G., Forbes, J., and Garraway, M. (1995). Interpreting self reported limiting long term illness. *British Medical Journal*, **311**, 722–4.

Cramer, D.W., Harlow, B.L., Willett, W.C., Welch, W.R., Bell, D.A., Scully, R.E., Ng, W.G., and Knapp, R.C. (1989). Galactose consumption and metabolism in relation to the risk of ovarian cancer. *Lancet*, **2**, 66–71.

Crum, J.E. (1993). Peak expiratory flow rate in schoolchildren living close to Braer oil spill. *British Medical Journal*, **307**, 23–4.

Daily Telegraph. (1999). London, 13 March, p. 9.

Damji, K.F., Shah, K.C., Rock, W.J., Bains, H.S., and Hodge, W.G. (1999). Selective laser trabeculoplasty v argon laser trabeculoplasty: a prospective randomised clinical trial. *British Journal of Ophthalmology*, **83**, 718–22.

Darby, S.C., Kendall, G.M., Fell, T.P., Doll, R., Goodill, A.A., Conquest, A.J., Jackson, D.A., and Haylock, R.G. (1993). Further follow up of mortality and incidence of cancer in men from the United Kingdom who participated in the United Kingdom's atmospheric nuclear weapon tests and experimental programmes. *British Medical Journal*, **307**, 1530–5.

Dennehy, J.A., Appleby, L., Thomas, C.S., and Faragher, E.B. (1996). Case–control study of suicide by discharged psychiatric patients. *British Medical Journal*, **312**, 1580.

DeStefano, F., Anda, R.F., Kahn, H.S., Williamson, D.F., and Russell, C.M. (1993). Dental disease and risk of coronary heart disease and mortality. *British Medical Journal*, **306**, 688–91.

Dickerson, J.E. and Brown, M.J. (1995). Influence of age on general practitioners' definition and treatment of hypertension. *British Medical Journal*, **310**, 574.

Dimitriou, G., Greenough, A., Kavvadia, V., Shute, M., and Karani, J. (1999). A radiographic method for assessing lung area in neonates. *British Journal of Radiology*, **72**, 335–8.

Eskenazi, B., Prehn, A.W., and Christianson, R.E. (1995). Passive and active maternal smoking as measured by serum cotinine: the effect on birthweight. *American Journal of Public Health*, **85**, 395–8.

Facchini, F.S., Hollenbeck, C.B., Jeppesen, J., Chen, Y.D., and Reaven, G.M. (1992). Insulin resistance and cigarette smoking. *Lancet*, **339**, 1128–30.

Fowkes, F.G. and Fulton, P.M. (1991). Critical appraisal of publication research: introductory guidelines. *British Medical Journal*, **302**, 1136–40.

Gaffney, G., Sellers, S., Flavell, V., Squier, M., and Johnson, A. (1994). Case–control study of intrapartum care, cerebral palsy, and perinatal death. *British Medical Journal*, **308**, 743–50.

Galloe, A.M., Rasmussen, H.S., Jorgensen, L.N., Aurup, P., Balslov, S., Cintin, C., Graudal, N., and McNair, P. (1993). Influence of oral magnesium supplementation on cardiac events among survivors of an acute myocardial infarction. *British Medical Journal*, **307**(6904), 585–7.

Gardner, M.J. (1989). Review of reported increases of childhood cancer rates in the vicinity of nuclear installations in the United Kingdom. *Journal of the Royal Statistical Society*, **152**, 307–25.

Gardosi, J., Hutson, N., and B-Lynch, C. (1989). Randomised, controlled trial of squatting in the second stage of labour. *Lancet*, **2**, 74–7.

Geelhoed, G.C., Turner, J., and Macdonald, W.B. (1996). Efficacy of a small single dose of oral dexamethasone for outpatient croup: a double blind placebo controlled clinical trial. *British Medical Journal*, **313**, 140–2.

Giles, G.G., Marks, R., and Foley, P. (1988). Incidence of non-melanocytic skin cancer treated in Australia. *British Medical Journal Clinical Research Ed*, **296**, 13–7.

Ginsburg, E.S., Mello, N.K., Mendelson, J.H., Barbieri, R.L., Teoh, S.K., Rothman, M., Gao, X., and Sholar, J.W. (1996). Effects of alcohol ingestion on estrogens in postmenopausal women. *JAMA*, **276**, 1747–51.

Gubitz, G. and Sandercock, P. (2000). Acute ischaemic stroke. *British Medical Journal*, **320**, 692–6.

Haddow, J.E., Knight, G.J., Paloaki, G.E., and McCarthy, J.E. (1988). Second trimester serum cotinine levels in nonsmokers in relation to birthweight. *American Journal of Obstetrics and Gynecology*, **159**, 481–4.

Hansard (1991). Referred to in *RSS News* (1992) **18**(7), 12

Harvey, J. and Prescott, R.J. (1994). Simple aspiration versus intercostal tube drainage for spontaneous pneumothorax in patients with normal lungs. *British Medical Journal*, **309**, 1338–9.

Hawthorne, V.M., Greaves, D.A., and Beevers, D.G. (1974). Blood pressure in a Scottish town. *British Medical Journal*, **3**, 600–3.

Haynes, J. and Hawkey, P.M. (1989). Providencia alcalifaciens and travellers' diarrhoea. *British Medical Journal*, **299**, 94–5.

Heathcote, J.A. (1995). Why do old men have big ears? *British Medical Journal*, **311**, 1668.

Helmstaedter, C. and Elger, C.E. (1999). The phantom of progressive dementia in epilepsy. *Lancet*, **354**, 2133–4.

Heywood, P. (1991). PACT level 3—a tool for audit. *Practitioner*, **235**, 450–1.

Hobbs, M., Mayou, R., Harrison, B., and Worlock, P. (1996). A randomised controlled trial of psychological debriefing for victims of road traffic accidents. *British Medical Journal*, **313**, 1438–9.

Hofman, A. and Walter, H.J. (1989). The association between physical fitness and cardiovascular disease risk factors in children in a five-year follow-up study. *International Journal of Epidemiology*, **18**, 830–5.

Holiday Which? (1999). Sick leave. Autumn issue.

Howie, J.G., Heaney, D.J., Maxwell, M., Walker, J.J., Freeman, G.K., and Rai, H. (1999). Quality at general practice consultations: cross sectional survey. *British Medical Journal*, **319**, 738–43.

Howie, P.W., Forsyth, J.S., Ogston, S.A., Clark, A., and Florey, C.D. (1990). Protective effect of breast feeding against infection. *British Medical Journal*, **300**, 11–6.

Jigjinni, V.S.S. (1997). The beefburger injury: a retrospective survey. *British Medical Journal*, **315**, 580.

Jones, C.M., Taylor, G.O., Whittle, J.G., Evans, D., and Trotter, D.P. (1997). Water fluoridation, tooth decay in 5 year olds, and social deprivation measured by the Jarman score: analysis of data from British dental surveys. *British Medical Journal*, **315**, 514–7

Kendall, M.G. (1970). *Rank Correlation Methods* 4th Ed., Griffin, London.

Kragballe, K., Gjertsen, B.T., De Hoop, D., Karlsmark, T., van de Kerkhof, P.C., Larko, O., Nieboer, C., Roed-Petersen, J., Strand, A., and Tikjob, G. (1991). Double-blind, right/left comparison of calcipotriol and betamethasone valerate in treatment of psoriasis vulgaris. *Lancet*, **337**, 193–6.

Lancet. (2000). Department of error – the phantom of progressive dementia in epilepsy. *Lancet*, **355**, 1020.

Larsson, K., Ohlsen, P., Larsson, L., Malmberg, P., Rydstrom, P.O., and Ulriksen, H. (1993). High prevalence of asthma in cross country skiers. *British Medical Journal*, **307**, 1326–9.

Lazzaroni, F., Bonassi, S., and Manniello, E. (1990). Effect of passive smoking during pregnancy on selected perinatal parameters. *International Journal of Epidemiology*, **19**, 960–5.

Lean, D. (1957). *The Bridge on the River Kwai*. Columbia Pictures.

Lentner, C. (1984). *Geigy Scientific Tables, Vol. 3*, Ciba-Geigy, Basle.

Leon, D.A., Koupilova, I., Lithell, H.O., Berglund, L., Mohsen, R., Vagero, D., Lithell, U.B., and McKeigue, P.M. (1996). Failure to realise growth potential *in utero* and adult obesity in relation to blood pressure in 50 year old Swedish men. *British Medical Journal*, **312**, 401–6.

Leung, S.F., Tsao, S.Y., Teo, P.M., Choi, P.H., and Shiu, W.C. (1991). Ovarian ablation failures by radiation: a comparison of two dose schedules. *British Journal of Radiology*, **64**, 537–8.

Lindberg, G., Eklund, G.A., Gullberg, B., and Rastam, L. (1991). Serum sialic acid concentration and cardiovascular mortality. *British Medical Journal*, **302**, 143–6.

Lucie, N.P. (1989). Radon exposure and leukaemia. *Lancet*, **2**, 99–100.

Lumb, A.B. and Vail, A. (2000). Difficulties with anonymous shortlisting of medical school applications and its effects on candidates with non-European names: prospective cohort study. *British Medical Journal*, **320**, 82–5.

Lund, M.B., Myhre, K.I., Melsom, H., and Johansen, B. (1991). The effect on pulmonary function of tangential field technique in radiotherapy for carcinoma of the breast. *British Journal of Radiology*, **64**, 520–3.

MacLennan, A.H., Wilson, D.H., and Taylor, A.W. (1996). Prevalence and cost of alternative medicine in Australia. *Lancet*, **347**, 569–73.

Maggiorini, M., Bartsch, P., and Oelz, O. (1997). Association between raised body temperature and acute mountain sickness: cross sectional study. *British Medical Journal*, **315**, 403–4.

Mainous, A.G. and Hueston, W.J. (1994). Passive smoking and low birth weight. Evidence of a threshold effect. *Archives of Family Medicine*, **3**, 875–8.

Malin, A., Ternouth, I., and Sarbah, S. (1994). Epitrochlear lymph nodes as marker of

HIV disease in sub-Saharan Africa. *British Medical Journal*, **309**, 1550–1.

Mann, R.E., Anglin, L., Wilkins, K., Vingilis, E., and MacDonald, S. (1993). Mortality in a sample of convicted drinking drivers. *Addiction*, **88**, 643–7.

Martin, T.R. and Bracken, M.B. (1986). Association of low birth weight with passive smoke exposure in pregnancy. *American Journal of Epidemiology*, **124**, 633–42.

Martinez, F.D., Wright, A.L., and Taussig, L.G. (1994). The effect of paternal smoking on the birthweight of newborns whose mothers did not smoke. *Public Health Briefs*, **84**, 1489–91.

Mathai, M., Vijayasri, R., Babu, S., and Jeyaseelan, L. (1992). Passive maternal smoking and birthweight in a South Indian Population. *British Journal of Obstetrics and Gynaecology*, **99**, 342–3.

McGarry, G.W., Gatehouse, S., and Hinnie, J. (1994). Relation between alcohol and nose bleeds. *British Medical Journal*, **309**, 640.

McKeeken, J., Stillman, B., Story, I., Kent, P., and Smith, J. (1999). The effects of knee extensor and flexor muscle training on the timed-up-and-go test in individuals with rheumatoid arthritis. *Physiotherapy Research International*, **4**, 55–67.

McMurdo, M.E., Mole, P.A., and Paterson, P.R. (1997). Controlled trial of weight bearing exercise in older women in relation to bone density and falls. *British Medical Journal*, **314**, 569.

Milne, S. (1999). Women find balancing work and family life 'increasingly arduous', says survey. *The Guardian*, London, 2 April, p.4.

Morabia, A. and Wynder, E.L. (1992). Relation of bronchioloalveolar carcinoma to tobacco. *British Medical Journal*, **304**, 541–3.

MRC Lung Cancer Working Party (1999). Treatment of endotracheal or endobronchial obstruction by non-small cell lung cancer: lack of patients in an MRC randomized trial leaves key questions unanswered. *Clinical Oncology*, **11**, 179–83.

Nott, M.R., Clemson, C.J., and Peacock, J.L. (1996). Onset time of topical analgesia with EMLA 5%: no reduction with glyceryl trinitrate. *European Journal of Anaesthesiology*, **13**, 17–20.

Ogawa, H., Tominaga, S., and Hori, K. (1991). Passive smoking by pregnant women and fetal growth. *Journal of Epidemiology and Community Health*, **45**, 164–8.

Oscier, D.G. (1997). ABC of clinical haematology. The myelodysplastic syndromes. *British Medical Journal*, **314**, 883–6.

Osterziel, K.J., Strohm, O., Schuler, J., Friedrich, M., Hänlein, D., Willenbrock, R., Anker, S.D., Poole-Wilson, P.A., Ranke, M.B., and Dietz, R. (1998). Randomised, double-blind, placebo-controlled trial of human recombiant growth hormone in patients with chronic heart failure due to dilated cardiomyopathy. *Lancet*, **351**, 1233–7.

Paradise, J.L., Bernard, B.S., Colborn, D.K., and Janosky, J. (1998). Assessment of adenoidal obstruction in children: clinical signs versus roentgenographic findings. *Pediatrics*, **101**, 979–86.

Paraskevaides, E.C., Pennington, G.W., Naik, S., and Gibbs, A.A. (1991). Prefreeze/post-freeze semen mortality ratio. *Lancet*, **337**, 366–7.

Pawlikowska, T., Chalder, T., Hirsch, S.R., Wallace, P., Wright, D.J.M., and Wessely.

S.C. (1994). Population based study of fatigue and psychological distress. *British Medical Journal*, **308**, 763–6.

Peacock, J.L. (1996). Endoscopic sphincterotomy with gall bladder left *in situ* versus open surgery for common bileduct calculi (letter). *Lancet*, **348**, 265.

Peacock, J.L., Bland, J.M., and Anderson, H.R. (1995). Preterm delivery: effects of socioeconomic factors, psychological stress, smoking, alcohol, and caffeine. *British Medical Journal*, **311**, 531–5.

Peacock, J.L., Cook, D.G., Carey, I.M., Jarvis, M.J., Bryant, A.E., Anderson, H.R., and Bland, J.M. (1998). Maternal cotinine level during pregnancy and birthweight for gestational age. *International Journal of Epidemiology*, **27**, 647–56.

Pearson, E.S. and Hartley H.O. (1972). *Biometrika Tables for Statisticians*, Cambridge University Press, Cambridge.

Penttinen, J. (1994). Back pain and risk of fatal ischaemic heart disease: 13 year follow up of Finnish farmers. *British Medical Journal*, **309**, 1267–8.

Peto, R., Gray, R., Collins, R., Wheatley, K., Hennekens, C., Jamrozik, K., Warlow, C., Hafner, B., Thompson, E., Norton, S., *et al.* (1988). Randomised trial of prophylactic daily aspirin in British male doctors. *British Medical Journal Clinical Research Ed*, **296**, 313–6.

Pettersson, E., Gardulf, A., Nordstrom, G., Svanberg-Johnsson, C., and Bylin, G. (1999). Evaluation of a nurse-run asthma school. *International Journal of Nursing Studies*, **36**, 145–51.

Peyrat, J.P., Bonneterre, J., Lubin, R., Vanlemmens, L., Fournier, J., and Soussi, T. (1995). Prognostic significance of circulating P53 antibodies in patients undergoing surgery for locoregional breast cancer. *Lancet*, **345**, 621–2.

Ponsonby, A.L., Dwyer, T., Gibbons, L.E., Cochrane, J.A., Jones, M.E., and McCall, M.J. (1992). Thermal environment and sudden infant death syndrome: case–control study. *British Medical Journal*, **304**, 277–82.

Prima Magazine (1999). We know the importance of family life. March issue, pp. 31–32.

Quinn, M.W., Wild, J., Dean, H.G., Hartley, R., Rushforth, J.A., Puntis, J.W., and Levene, M.I. (1993). Randomised double-blind controlled trial of effect of morphine on catecholamine concentrations in ventilated pre-term babies. *Lancet*, **342**, 324–7.

Rafferty, T., Wilson-Davis, K., and McGavock, H. (1997). How has fundholding in Northern Ireland affected prescribing patterns? A longitudinal study. *British Medical Journal*, **315**, 166–70.

Reid, I.R., Chin, K., Evans, M.C., and Jones, J.G. (1994). Relation between increase in length of hip axis in older women between 1950s and 1990s and increase in age specific rates of hip fracture. *British Medical Journal*, **309**, 508–9.

Rennie, A.N. (1997). Prevalence of arm movements in patients with coronary heart disease: case–control study. *British Medical Journal*, **314**, 122.

Richardson, J., Stratford, P., and Cripps, D. (1998). Assessment of reliability of the hand-held dynamometer for measuring strength in healthy older adults. *Physiotherapy Theory and Practice*, **14**, 49–54.

Riemersma, R.A., Wood, D.A., Macintyre, C.C., Elton, R.A., Gey, K.F., and Oliver, M.F. (1991). Risk of angina pectoris and plasma concentrations of vitamins A, C, and E and carotene. *Lancet*, **337**, 1-5.

Rivellese, A.A., Auletta, P., Marotta, G., Saldalamacchia, G., Giacco, A., Mastrilli, V., Vaccaro, O., and Riccardi, G. (1994). Long term metabolic effects of two dietary methods of treating hyperlipidaemia. *British Medical Journal*, **308**, 227-31.

Rookus, M.A. and van Leeuwen, F.E. (1994). Oral contraceptives and risk of breast cancer in women aged 20-54 years. Netherlands Oral Contraceptives and Breast Cancer Study Group. *Lancet*, **344**, 844-51.

RSS News (1999). Forsooth. June issue.

Rubin, D.H., Krasilnikoff, P.A., Leventhal, J.M., Weile, P.A., and Berget, A. (1986). Effect of passive smoking on birthweight. *Lancet*, **ii**, 415-7.

Sackett, D.L., Haynes, R.B., Guyatt, G.H., and Tugwell, P. (1991). *Clinical Epidemiology: A Basic Science for Clinical Medicine*, Little, Brown, Boston.

Salvesen, K.A., Bakketeig, L.S., Eik-nes, S.H., Undheim, J.O., and Okland, O. (1992). Routine ultrasonography *in utero* and school performance. *Lancet*, **339**, 85-9.

Sanci, L.A., Coffey, C.M., Veit, F.C., Carr-Gregg, M., Patton, G.C., Day, N., and Bowes, G. (2000). Evaluation of the effectiveness of an educational intervention for general practitioners in adolescent health care: randomised controlled trial. *British Medical Journal*, **320**, 224-30.

Schwartz, L.M., Woloshin, S., Black, W.C., and Welch, H.G. (1997). The role of numeracy in understanding the benefit of screening mammography. *Annals of Internal Medicine*, **127**, 966-72.

Sharma, S.D., Smith, E.M., Hazleman, B.L., and Jenner, J.R. (1997). Thermographic changes in keyboard operators with chronic forearm pain. *British Medical Journal*, **314**, 118.

Sharpe, M., Hawton, K., Simkin, S., Surawy, C., Hackmann, A., Klimes, I., Peto, T., and Warrell, D. (1996). Cognitive behaviour therapy for the chronic fatigue syndrome: a randomized controlled trial. *British Medical Journal*, **312**, 22-6.

Sherman, D.I., Ward, R.J., Warren-Perry, M., Williams, R., and Peters, T.J. (1993). Association of restriction fragment length polymorphism in alcohol dehydrogenase 2 gene with alcohol induced liver damage. *British Medical Journal*, **307**, 1388-90.

Singh, B.M., Prescott, J.J., Guy, R., Walford, S., Murphy, M., and Wise, P.H. (1994). Effect of advertising on awareness of symptoms of diabetes among the general public: the British Diabetic Association Study. *British Medical Journal*, **308**, 632-6.

Smith, J. and Channer, K.S. (1995). Increasing prescription of drugs for secondary prevention after myocardial infarction. *British Medical Journal*, **311**, 917-8.

Smith, M. (1980). Will it happen again? *Women's Own* June issue.

Spector, T.D., Cicuttini, F., Baker, J., Loughlin, J., and Hart, D. (1996). Genetic influences on osteoarthritis in women: a twin study. *British Medical Journal*, **312**, 940-3.

Spence, D.P., Hotchkiss, J., Williams, C.S., and Davies, P.D. (1993). Tuberculosis and poverty. *British Medical Journal*, **307**, 759-61.

St. George, D. (1986). Life expectancy, truth, and the ABPI. *Lancet*, **2**, 346.

Stell, I.M. and Gransden, W.R. (1998). Simple tests for septic bursitis: comparitive study. *British Medical Journal*, **316**, 1877.

Stoeber, K., Halsall, I., Freeman, A., Swinn, R., Doble, A., Morris, L., Coleman, N., Bullock, N., Laskey, R.A., Hales, C.N., and Williams, G.H. (1999). Immunoassay for urothelial cancers that detects DNA replication protein Mcm5 in urine. *Lancet*, **354**, 1524–5.

Taddio, A., Goldbach, M., Ipp, M., Stevens, B., and Koren, G. (1995). Effect of neonatal circumcision on pain responses during vaccination in boys. *Lancet*, **345**, 291–2.

Talbot (1999). Positively false on HIV. *The Guardian*, London, 28 September, p.21.

Tan, L.B. (1997). New method for expressing survival in cancer. Use of percentage of 'normal remaining life' may be confusing. *British Medical Journal*, **315**, 1375.

Targarona, E.M., Ayuso, R.M., Bordas, J.M., Ros, E., Pros, I., Martinez, J., Teres, J., and Trias, M. (1996a). Randomised trial of endoscopic sphincterotomy with gallbladder left *in situ* versus open surgery for common bileduct calculi in high-risk patients. *Lancet*, **347**, 926–9.

Targarona, E.M., Perez Ayuso, R.M., Ros, E., Teres, J., and Trias, M. (1996b). Endoscopic sphincterotomy with gall bladder left *in situ* versus open surgery for common bileduct calculi—authors' reply. *Lancet*, **348**, 265.

Taylor, J.C., Norman, C.L., Bland, J.M., Ramsey, J.D., and Anderson, H.R. (1999). Trends in deaths associated with abuse of volatile substances 1971–1997: Report no. 12. St. George's Hospital Medical School, London.

ten Wolde, S., Breedveld, F.C., Hermans, J., Vandenbroucke, J.P., van de Laa, M.A., Markusse, H.M., Janssen, M., van den Brink, H.R., and Dijkmans, B.A. (1996). Randomised placebo-controlled study of stopping second-line drugs in rheumatoid arthritis. *Lancet*, **347**, 347–52.

The Guardian (1998). Consumer: Why can't I find trousers with waist sizes measured in odd numbers? London, 28 May, p.17.

The Guardian (1999). Gould takes on his critics. London, 31 August, p.23.

The Mirror (1999). 20 million-to-1 family. London, 28 January, p.3.

Tonnesen, H., Rosenberg, J., Nielsen, H.J., Rasmussen, V., Hauge, C., Pedersen, Ib.K., and Kehlet, H. (1999). Effect of preoperative abstinence on poor postoperative outcome in alcohol misusers: randomised controlled trial. *British Medical Journal*, **318**, 1311–6.

Tsushima, Y., Tamura, T., Tomioka, K., Okada, C., Kusano, S., and Endo, K. (1999). Transient splenomegaly in acute pancreatitis. *British Journal of Radiology*, **72**, 637–43.

Turnbull, D., Holmes, A., Shields, N., Cheyne, H., Twaddle, S., Gilmour, W.H., McGinley, M., Reid, M., Johnstone, I., Geer, I., McIlwaine, G., and Lunan, C.B. (1996). Randomised, controlled trial of efficacy of midwife-managed care. *Lancet*, **348**, 213–8.

Vaidya, J.S. and Mittra, I. (1997). Fraction of normal remaining life span: a new method for expressing survival in cancer. *British Medical Journal*, **314**, 1682–4.

Vaidya, J.S. and Mittra, I. (1998). New method of expressing survival in cancer is popular. *British Medical Journal*, **316**, 1092.

Varghese, Z., Scoble, J.E., Chan, M.K., Wheeler, D., Lui, S.F., Baillod, R.A., Fernado, O.N., Sweny, P., and Moorhead, J.F. (1988). Parathyroid hormone as a causative factor of primary non-function in renal transplants. *British Medical Journal*, **296**, 393.

Vartiainen, E., Puska, P., Pekkanen, J., Tuomilehto, J., Lonnqvist, J., Ehnholm, and C. (1994). Serum cholesterol concentration and mortality from accidents, suicide, and other violent causes. *British Medical Journal*, **309**, 445–7.

Verdrager, J. (1998). New variant Creutzfeldt-Jakob disease and bovine pituitary growth hormone. *Lancet*, **351**, 112–3.

Wallace, S.J. and Smith, J.A. (1980). Successful prophylaxis against febrile convulsions with valproic acid or phenobarbitone. *British Medical Journal*, **280**, 353–4.

Ward, H., Day, S., Mezzone, J., Dunlop, L., Donegan, C., Farrar, S., Whitaker, L., Harris, J.R., and Miller, D.L. (1993). Prostitution and risk of HIV: female prostitutes in London. *British Medical Journal*, **307**, 356–8.

Webb, P.M., Knight, T., Greaves, S., Wilson, A., Newell, D.G., Elder, J., and Forman, D. (1994). Relation between infection with *Helicobacter pylori* and living conditions in childhood: evidence for person to person transmission in early life. *British Medical Journal*, **308**, 750–3.

Weissman, M.M., Klerman, G.L., Markowitz, J.S., and Ouellette, R. (1989). Suicidal ideation and suicide attempts in panic disorder and attacks. *New England Journal of Medicine*, **321**, 1209–14.

West, K.P., Katz, J., Khatry, S.K., LeClerq, S.C., Pradhan, E.K., Shrestha, S.R., Connor, P.B., Dali, S.M., Christian, P., Pokhrel, R.P., and Sommer, A. (1999). Double blind, cluster randomised trial of low dose supplementation with vitamin A or beta-carotene on mortality related to pregnancy in Nepal. *British Medical Journal*, **318**, 570–5.

West, M.J., Coleman, P.D., Flood, D.G., and Troncoso, J.C. (1994). Differences in the pattern of hippocampal neuronal loss in normal ageing and Alzheimer's disease. *Lancet*, **344**, 769–72.

Whitley, E., Gunnell, D., Dorling, D., and Smith, G.D. (1999). Ecological study of social fragmentation, poverty, and suicide. *British Medical Journal*, **319**, 1034–7.

Wilkinson, C.E., Peters, T.J., Stott, N.C., and Harvey, I.M. (1994). Prospective evaluation of a risk scoring system for cervical neoplasia in primary care. *British Journal of General Practice*, **44**, 341–4.

Wilkinson, R., Milledge, J.S., and Landon, M.J. (1993). Microalbuminuria in chronic obstructive lung disease. *British Medical Journal*, **307**, 239.

Wilkinson, R.G. (1992). Income distribution and life expectancy. *British Medical Journal*, **304**, 165–8.

Winters, J.C., Sobel, J.S., Groenier, K.H., Arendzen, H.J., and Meijboom-de Jong, B. (1997). Comparison of physiotherapy, manipulation and corticosteroid injection for treating shoulder complaints in general practice: randomised, single blind study. *British Medical Journal*, **314**, 1320–5.

Winters, J.C., Jorritsma, W., Groenier, K.H., Sobel, J.S., and Meijboom-de Jong, B. (1999). Treatment of shoulder complaints in general practice: long term results of a randomised, single blind study comparing physiotherapy, manipulation, and corticosteroid injection. *British Medical Journal*, **318**, 1395–6.

Wise, J. (1998). Links to tobacco industry influences review conclusions. *British Medical Journal*, **316**, 1533.

Wjst, M., Reitmeir, P., Dold, S., Wulff, A., Nicolai, T., von, Loeffelholz-Colberg, E.F., and von Mutius, E. (1993). Road traffic and adverse effects on respiratory health in children. *British Medical Journal*, **307**, 596–600.

Wood, A. (1999). Exclusion orders: for and against. *The Guardian*, London, 3 September, p.19.

Zhang, J. and Radcliffe, J.M. (1993). Paternal smoking and birthweight in Shanghi. *American Journal of Public Health*, **83**, 207–10.